M000105525

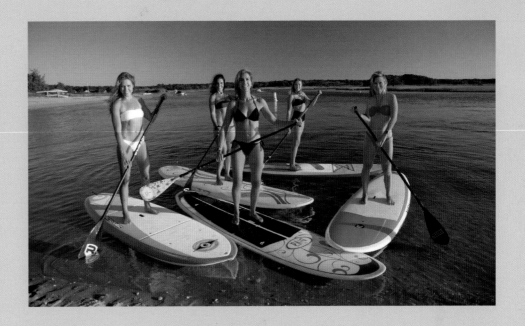

"It was so peaceful and meditative to be on the water and in rhythm with nature once I started to get the hang of it. It certainly helps when you have a guide like Gina Bradley who makes even challenging conditions look effortless. I learned in this practice that beauty is balance and balance is beauty."

—CHRISTY TURLINGTON BURNS, Founder of Every Mother Counts

"Gina Bradley has taught me how to enjoy being on the water and to take each stroke on a paddleboard with mindfulness. She exudes positivity and her Guiding Principles encourage people on their journey in life to feel balanced and beautiful, and to celebrate Nature's wonders."

—SUSAN ROCKEFELLER

"Having the chance to spend time with Gina on the paddleboards was bliss. Besides the super instruction, Gina gave us a great insight into the natural habitat. Every session on the board was a rewarding experience."

—NADJA SWAROVSKI-ADAMS

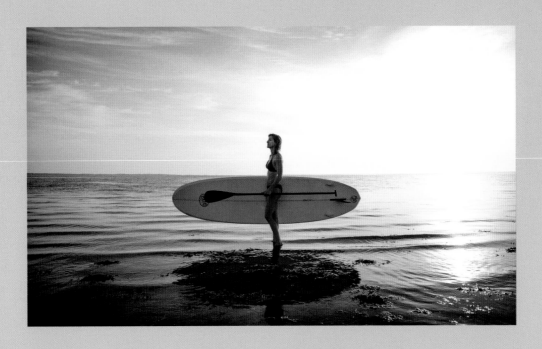

PADDLE DIVA

Ten Guiding Principles to Finding Balance on the Water and in Life

GINA BRADLEY

Post Hill
PRESS

A POST HILL PRESS BOOK

Paddle Diva:
Ten Guiding Principles to Finding Balance on the Water and in Life
© 2019 by Gina Bradley
All Rights Reserved

ISBN: 978-1-64293-135-8

Cover design by Bill Bonnell
Cover photo by Michael Williams
Interior design and composition by Greg Johnson, Textbook Perfect

No part of this book may be reproduced, stored in a retrieval system, or transmitted
by any means without the written permission of the author and publisher.

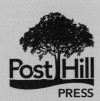

Post Hill Press
New York • Nashville
posthillpress.com

Published in the United States of America
Printed in China

To Scott, James, and Emma,

who have tested my truth

in every principle

at one point or another.

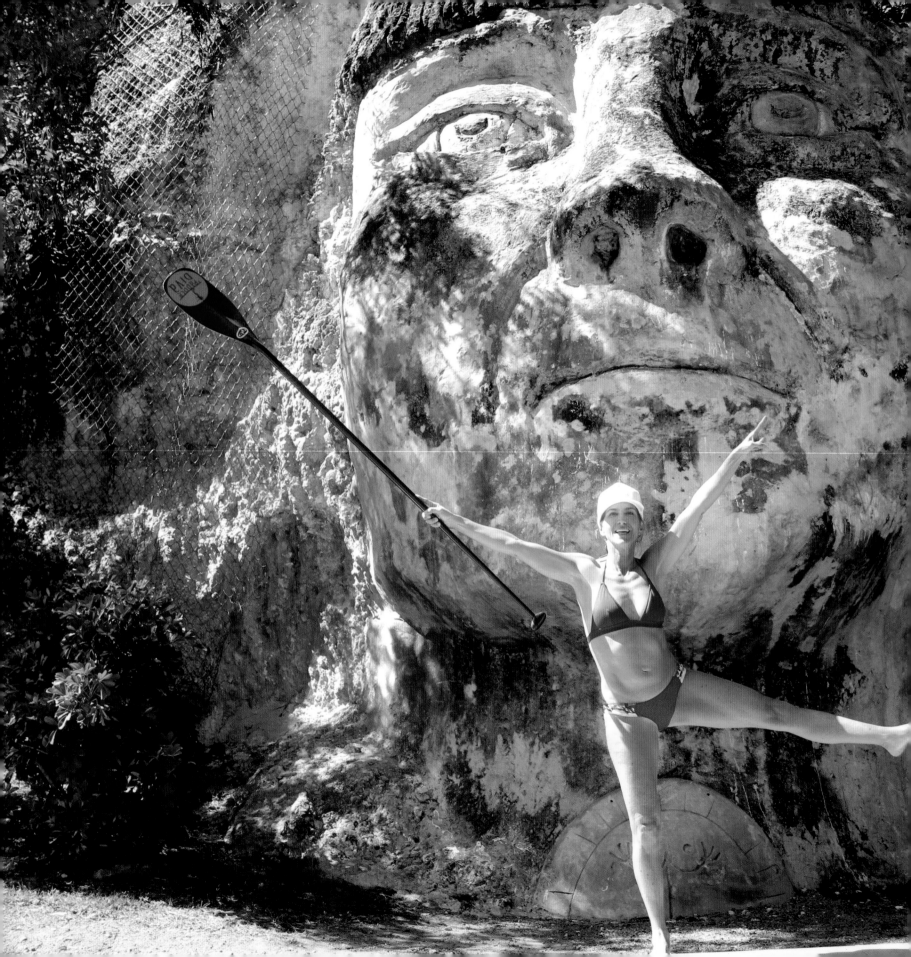

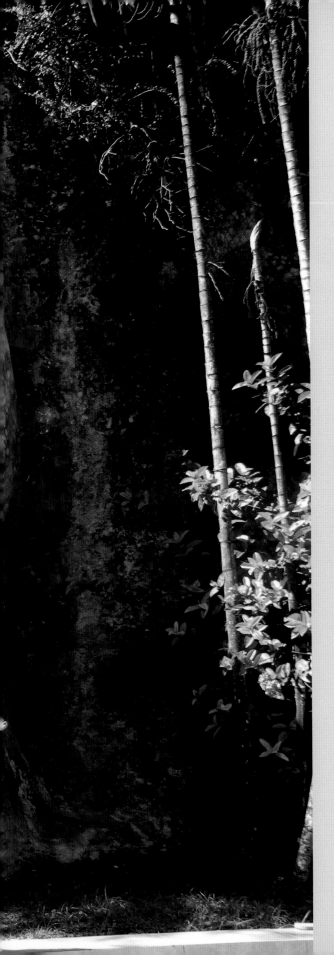

Contents

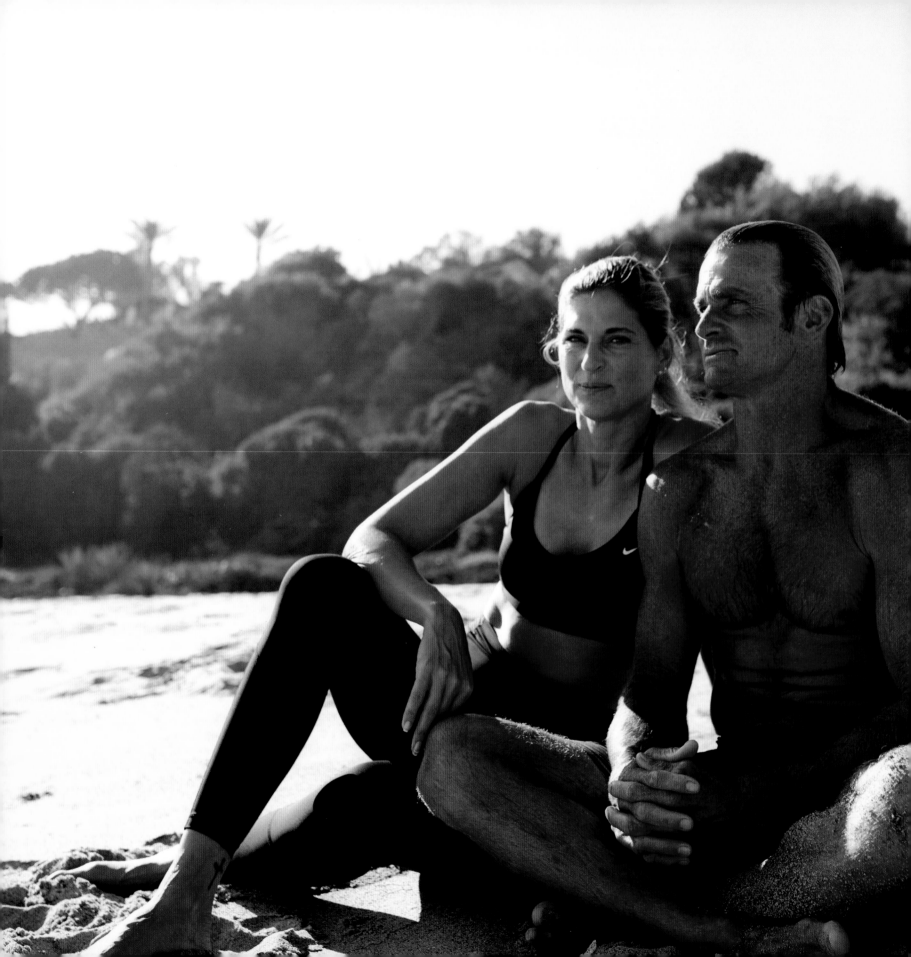

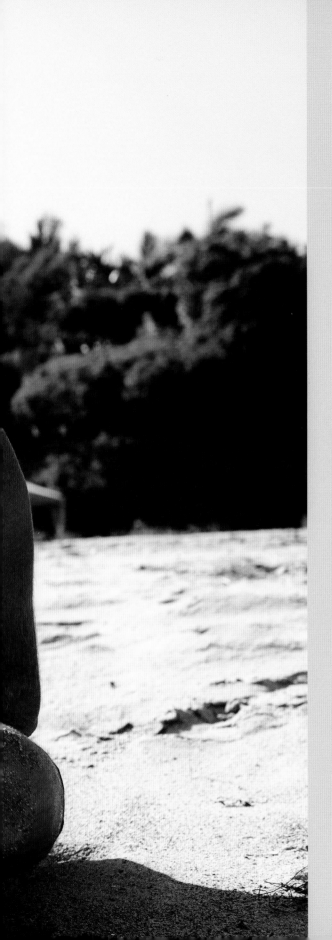

Foreword

When we first pulled up to the Paddle Diva Center East Hampton in 2016, we were greeted by Gina Bradley and quickly understood how, in the seven years since she founded her stand-up paddleboard company, she had made such a foothold in the sport on the East Coast. She's the perfect infusion of energy and positivity and has the capacity to get a lot done in a way that appears effortless. If we have learned one thing, it's that the easier someone makes it look the better they are at spinning all the plates.

Finding balance and adapting in life is something we all strive for. We do it every day, from the moment we wake till we finally rest when the sun goes down. As much as we are in sync with one another, we each approach this so very differently. One of us heads to the ocean in search of balance and the other finds it in exercise, work, and keeping the beat of the household going. While we go to different places, we are both looking for the same release, the same sense of calm, balance, and perspective to keep us composed as we move through life. Our days seem busy to an outside observer (and they are), but we are both anchors to one another as we hold firm in the massive seas that surround us. We use our physicality and learning as a way to connect to each other and those around us.

This is one of our common languages and as a natural extension of that we created our program XPT (Extreme Performance Training), an approach to a performance lifestyle that is rooted in the most basic yet powerful human trait: the ability to adapt. This program allows us to share what we know and what we have learned with our own students, and it gives them the opportunity to glide through life, adapting and finding balance.

As we paddled with our group of trainees during the Montauk XPT program that summer, we both knew immediately we had a new connection to the East Coast. Later, while hosting our dear friend Maria Baum's Hamptons Party and Paddle for Pink SUP race, we watched Gina cross the finish line and knew we were in the presence of someone who loves the marine environment. Like us, she is passionate about the ocean, moving in it or on it, working with it, and most clearly, finding balance in her life because of it. Gina possesses the ability to flow in and out of all sides of her personality. Loving and supportive, inviting, playful, curious, strong and with a kick-ass fighting spirit.

Whatever ocean you are near, the one thing we all have in common is that we are connected to the water. We are hatched in it, we bathe in it, we are composed mostly of it, and some of us, like Laird, play in it. For all of us, the key to living a balanced life is to stay fit mentally, emotionally, and physically. We are just trying to do our best as good examples in fitness with the hope of motivating and inspiring humans to be their best and perform to their fullest potential. It's this sort of mentality that connects all of us who strive for balance in our lives.

In the pages of this book, Gina offers you a window into the breathtaking views that can only be seen from the water and outlines her Ten Principles of Balance that integrate SUP fitness with personal empowerment. Use them as a roadmap to finding balance on the water and in life, so that you can rise up on your board and unleash the athlete within.

—Gabby Reece and Laird Hamilton

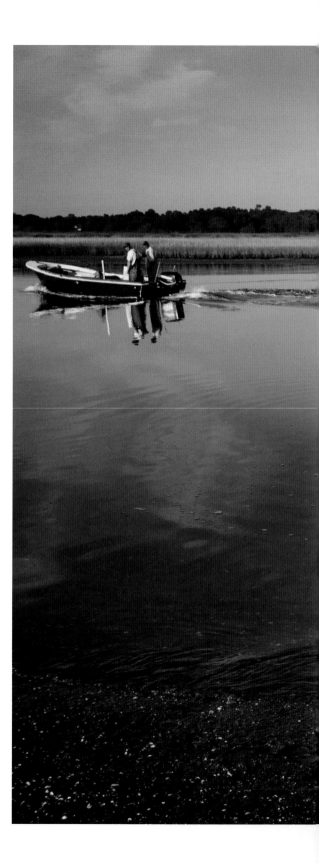

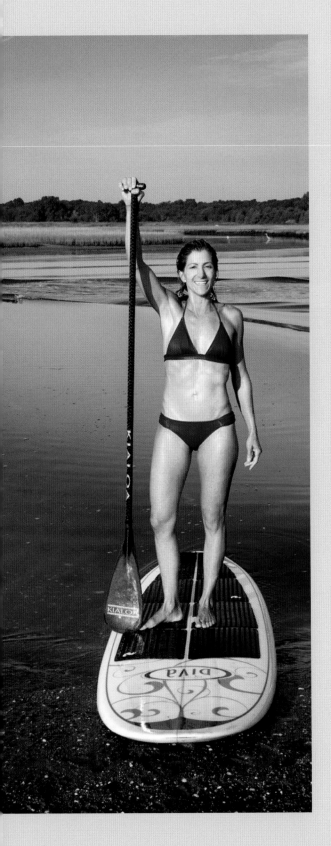

Introduction

My name is Gina Bradley, founder of Paddle Diva, a stand-up paddleboard (SUP) business that teaches women (and men) how to rise up on their paddleboards and in their lives. I opened my first center in the Hamptons, my home base, over ten years ago when the sport was in its infancy. Since then, Paddle Diva has become a household name, and my cozy marina waterfront location an iconic destination. It's a place that's on every resident's and vacationer's must-do list. As a recognized pioneer and current leader in my sport, I love working with my community both as a SUP instructor and as an advocate for our oceans.

Mention my name to a SUP enthusiast or local resident of the Hamptons and you will invariably hear how Paddle Diva has made a positive impact in their life. Meeting fellow adventure lovers who want to embrace the magic of SUP is what I love to do. If you are anywhere near one of our Paddle Diva centers, always feel welcome to stop by, say hi, share the your adventures, and join the tribe.

Aside from it being a really fun, full-body workout that anyone can master in just one hour, people are drawn to SUP—and Paddle Diva specifically—because of the transformation they see in their bodies and in their lives once

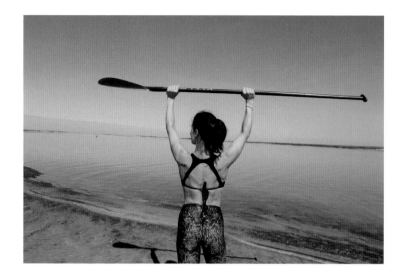

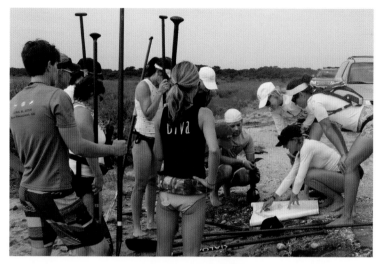

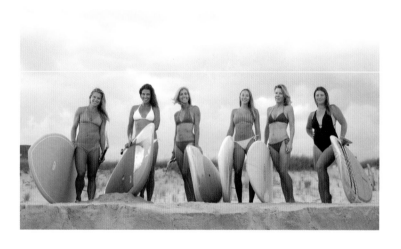

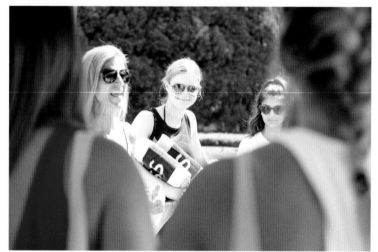

they give it a try. I've seen paddlers shed pounds, rebuild their strength after an illness or a pregnancy, overcome their fear of the water, forge unbreakable bonds with fellow paddlers, and—most important—take what they've learned on the water and apply it to their everyday lives. Paddle Divas live life to the fullest. We don't just sit on the shore and watch the water move; we move *with* the water. We come from a place of abundance, we laugh out loud, and we feel empowered by each stroke we take on our boards as we effortlessly glide through the water.

We Paddle Divas are a tribe of our own. We are a community of like-minded souls. When I meet someone who tells me they "love paddling," I know immediately we share many things in common. It's like a secret handshake. We know things that those who have not adventured out on a SUP will never know. When we paddle, we bring the freedom and energy that we feel on the water back to land and apply Paddle Diva's Ten Guiding Principles of Balance that move us forward on our boards to every other part of our lives.

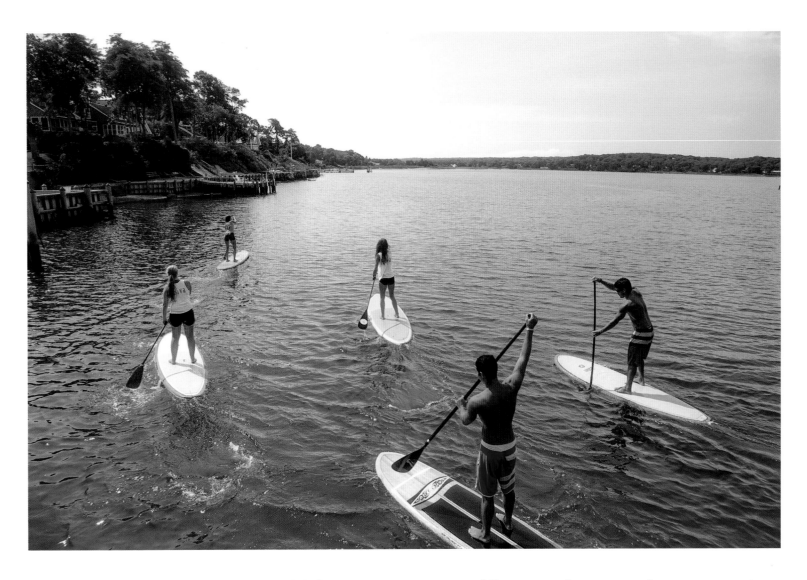

These principles, which I developed while learning SUP and carving out my ideal life, stretch from the water into every aspect of a Diva's world. They create an easy framework to shift our behavior from thought to action. I know because I live the Diva lifestyle every day. You could say that as one of the first mainstream proponents of this newly emerging sport, and the first to find a way to market it and make it accessible to all, I am the original Paddle Diva.

At Paddle Diva we don't just teach SUP; we promise a way of life. This book is a celebration of the women and men who are already immersed in our fast-growing community, as well as a window for newcomers into the transformational Paddle Diva lifestyle. Anyone can use these principles. SUP is practiced on the water, but the Paddle Diva approach to a happier, healthier, and better-balanced life exists everywhere.

Before I get too far ahead of myself, let's first talk about SUP and why it's so popular. For many, it feels like it's a

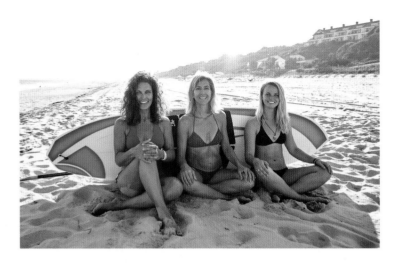
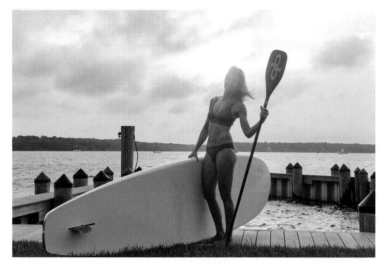
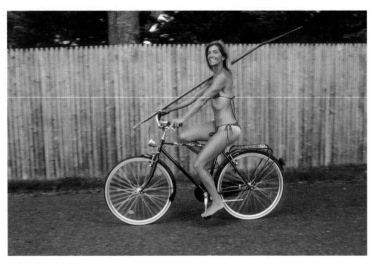
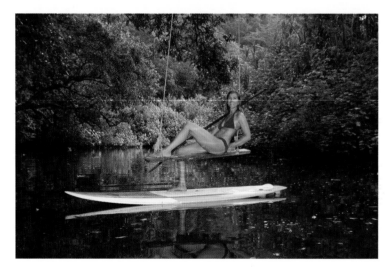

new sport that has gained tremendous popularity incredibly quickly. Why is that? For starters, it's a head-to-toe workout. Every time you stand on your board and place your paddle blade into the water and pull back, you fire up your abs and core muscles. You also engage your balance muscles—legs and hips—and, of course, your biceps and triceps come into play. While this may sound complicated, every first-timer is surprised by just how easy SUP is to learn and how magical it is to walk on water.

Variations on SUP date back thousands of years from many pockets around the globe. As we know it today, the sport was born out of Hawaiian surfing culture. SUP became popular thanks to Laird Hamilton, my friend and a surfing legend, who retrofitted a canoe paddle and a tandem surfboard to surf on small-wave days. Following September 11th, Laird was photographed paddling in Malibu, California, holding up the American flag, bringing SUP to the eyes of mainstream USA.

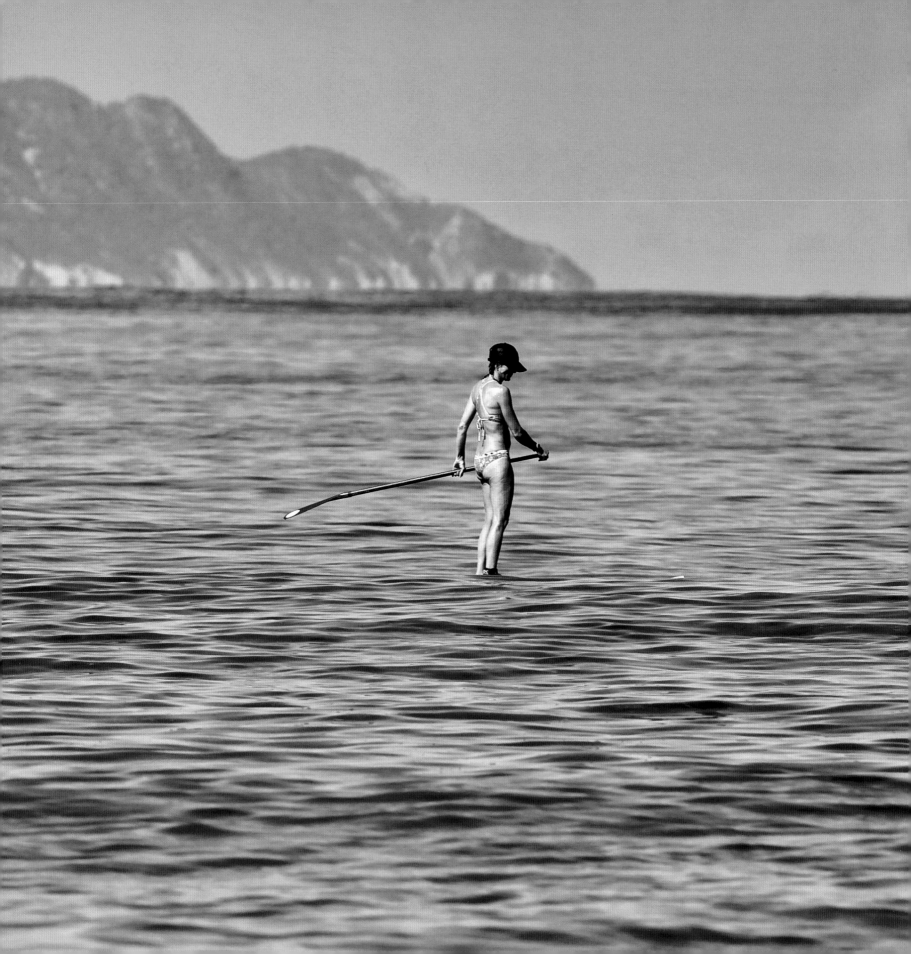

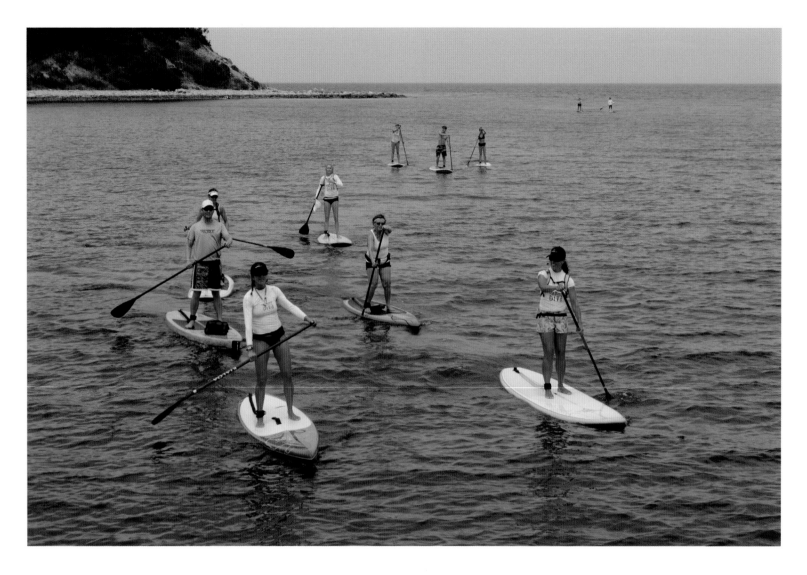

If you have not yet heard of or tried SUP, you stand ashore in a shrinking population. With its meteoric mainstream growth, SUP has captured the attention of the larger world of sports and fitness. The market for SUP clothing was non-existent when Paddle Diva first opened; now there is a wide choice of major brands offering workout wear specific to paddling. Television advertisements for everything from cars to medications to vacations feature brightly colored SUP boards with people smiling on top of them. Along every coastline or waterway, it's common now to see a silhouette moving gracefully along the horizon. It feels like SUP is everywhere, and it really is! Races, competitions, expositions, trade shows, and SUP shops have become commonplace throughout the world.

In step with the growth of the sport, the Paddle Diva movement is also on the rise. In ten years we've expanded from operating out of the back of a single pickup truck to having multiple locations on some of the most beautiful waters in the world. Along the way, Paddle Diva has

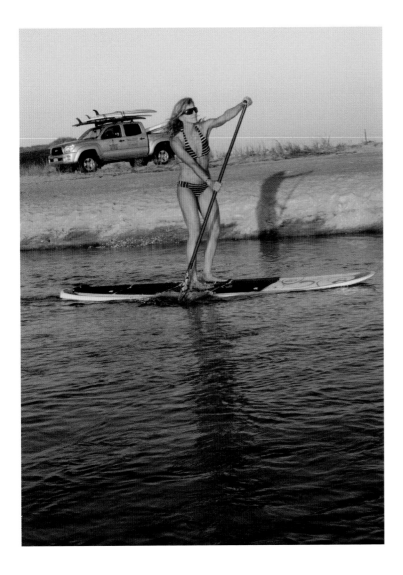

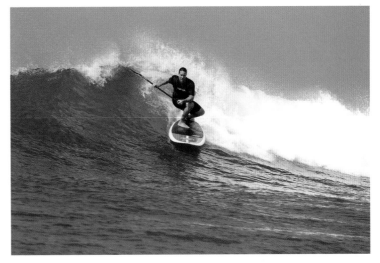

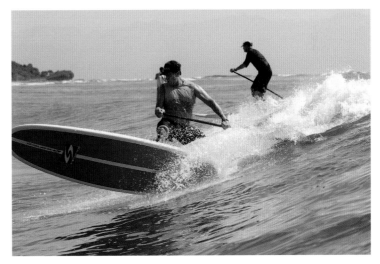

quickly become synonymous with the natural beauty of the Hamptons and its celebrity population. With Paddle Diva centers in the Shagwong Marina on Three Mile Harbor, East Hampton; a presence at the Surf Lodge and Gurney's in Montauk; the Waldorf Astoria's Boca Beach Club; and a beachfront location in Rincón, Puerto Rico, along with plans to be on Bermuda's Sinky Bay Beach, we are spreading our gospel of balance far and wide. My goal is for people around the world to have access to safe, fun, and reliable paddling, all while learning to take the Paddle Diva's Guiding Principles back to their lives onshore and unlock their full potential in all they do.

I began my own journey with the sport in 2009. As a fitness instructor, former windsurfing professional, and Professional Association of Diving Instructors–certified scuba instructor, I am always on the lookout for new ways to exercise outdoors, especially on the water. When my husband had a stand-up paddleboard custom built by our board shaper and friend Mike Becker of Nature Shapes, I decided to try SUP for myself. The very first

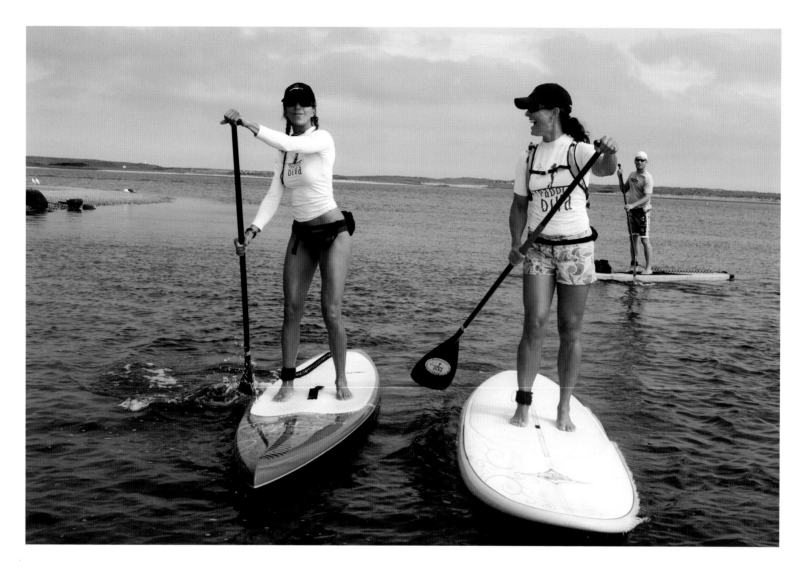

time I stood on a board and started paddling, I knew that I had found my passion. Yet, as with most watersports (think surfing and kite boarding), the early culture was predominantly masculine. The boards were huge and hard to carry, and you were required to paddle into the ocean, where you had to deal with the surf and rolling waves. All of the photos I saw were of men looking so intense and focused on their boards!

Women were most certainly underserved by the way the sport was developing, despite the fact that it was perfect for women's unique athletic strengths. One day, while I was paddling with two girlfriends, it occurred to me that SUP needed to have a place in the Hamptons—actually, the world! Women would love SUP if it were introduced to them in the right way. Through the crowd of guys standing up on their boards, I had a vision of a strong-looking female silhouette, commanding the board and standing on the water while the water rushed behind her. The seeds of Paddle Diva had been planted.

I started teaching SUP to my girlfriends in East Hampton and quickly found that it served as both a workout and a way for us to bond with one another while disconnecting from the stresses in our daily lives. Out on the water, we were free from the noise and clutter of the day and got to appreciate a new perspective of the world as we looked back at land. For the first time in a long time, these women relaxed (which is necessary in order to paddle effectively) and really opened up to one another about what was going on in their lives and what they wanted next—all while getting into shape. It was then that Paddle Diva was born.

In the weeks and months that followed, I developed a method that allowed me to teach women (regardless of body shape, size, weight, or fitness level) how to SUP successfully in *only one hour*. I designed new boards that were smaller and easier for women to carry and maneuver. I highlighted the transformational aspects of this sport—from the physical to the emotional. I began taking women out on the calm, sleepy bays of the east end of Long Island. As enrollment in my classes and private lessons climbed, SUP began to spread to women across the country and the globe.

What is it that Divas experience while paddling that they take back to land and use in their everyday lives? How do they transform what they learn on the water into the fuel that powers their dreams into reality, expands their limits, and urges them to live their best lives?

With a light voice and simple cues from me, you would get into a tabletop position and then look up and focus on a mark on the horizon. "You got this!" I'd reassure you as you stand up, smiling and probably holding your breath. I'd remind you to breathe in and then out,

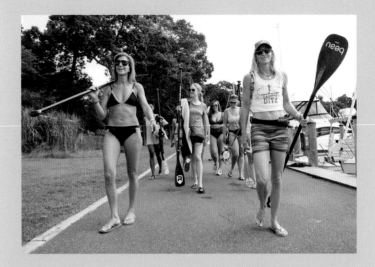

Here's What a Typical Paddle Diva Transformation Looks Like

We meet at the shop. My little ten-pound white rescue pup, Coconut, will sleepily greet you while resting on the counter, managing customer service. If it's your first time, you may be nervous and worried you won't be able to stand up. I will tell you that I have yet to be "broken" and that whoever paddles with me succeeds and stands. It's what we do here at Paddle Diva. We have all the teaching skill and experience to turn a novice into a pro.

As we chat on our way down to the water, the vibe will always be positive. At Paddle Diva, we set the stage with an infectious energy. As your teacher, I have already assumed you have succeeded as we walk down to the boards and put our leashes on. In about five minutes, I take you through what you need to know: how to hold the paddle; the proper position, stance, and paddle stroke; how to start by kneeling; how to stand and steer; and most important, how to fall off the board (which actually almost never happens). As you place your board in knee-deep water to start and kneel in the center—the sweet spot, as we call it—you can immediately feel how supportive these boards are as you start to paddle in this kneeling position.

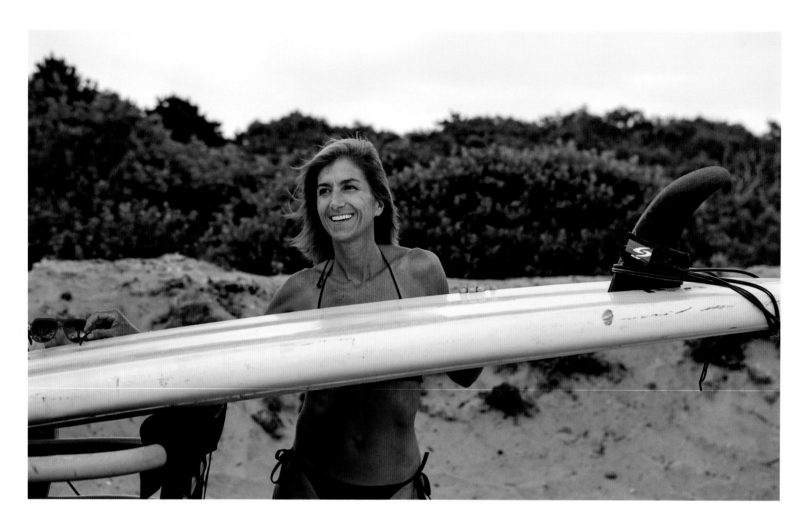

and your shoulders would relax. You are paddling. We are now on our journey, paddling and talking while I make simple corrections. As you gain confidence and control, you are well on your way to feeling like you can do anything from this day forward!

As our paddle continues, we work with your stroke so you really get the most dynamic workout possible. I encourage you to dig the paddle deep into the water on one side, then the other. As you start to really experiment with the "catch" or the plunge of your paddle into the water and your body leans into the power of the stroke, your core starts to engage. You may think, *Yes, I feel this in my core. I am getting it!* The wind would gently blow through your hair and you'd take in the beautiful landscape from your new vantage point. We'd both smile as I teach you the Diva 180, a stroke (whose name I coined) to turn your board around so you can head back to shore. I'd smile as I watch you turn back to land, realizing how far you have come in just a short amount of time. As we paddle together along the clear waters of the bay, I'd see you transforming. You would paddle back to shore a new person. You would feel relaxed. You would feel strong. You would feel empowered. You'd tell me how freeing it feels to *walk on water*.

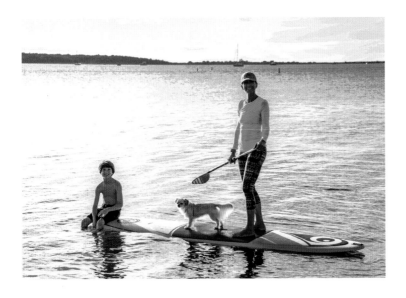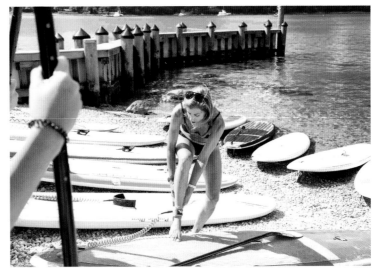

When our lesson ends and we walk back up to the office to rinse our feet and grab a cool drink, I would encourage you to take this new sense of energy and freedom back to your life. As you drive away, you would recall the many Guiding Principles we went over on the water and begin to think through where you can apply these to the parts of your life where you feel stuck and unbalanced. Maybe you would better connect with your family or a friend, even if just for that afternoon. Maybe you would be inspired to think more about eating a balanced diet and to drink plenty of water. Perhaps you'd sign up for that class you've been meaning to try. Best of all, within a few weeks of your doing SUP as your *only* exercise three times a week, your body would feel lighter, your abs firmer, and your life larger and more enjoyable. You would set goals and actually work towards them. You would begin by taking small steps towards change that would ultimately lead to a lifelong commitment to fitness, a healthy diet, and wellness, so that whenever the water calls, you will be ready to paddle out.

As the Paddle Diva movement builds momentum and ever-increasing numbers of new Divas are rising up on their boards and embracing our Guiding Principles, their confidence, physical strength, and sense of community soar. The water is calling to us, and there are endless possibilities for exploration and growth as we answer her call and step onto our boards. We have been given a life to live, and we are lucky to have a brand-new day that we can choose to enjoy to the fullest. This is the Paddle Diva way: we find balance on our boards, and we take it into our lives so we live the best lives ever! These principles will be your new guide, like a lighthouse guiding you back to land. I promise you will flourish, you will grow, you will be happy. Want to paddle? It's that easy. Come on, step on, and let's go!

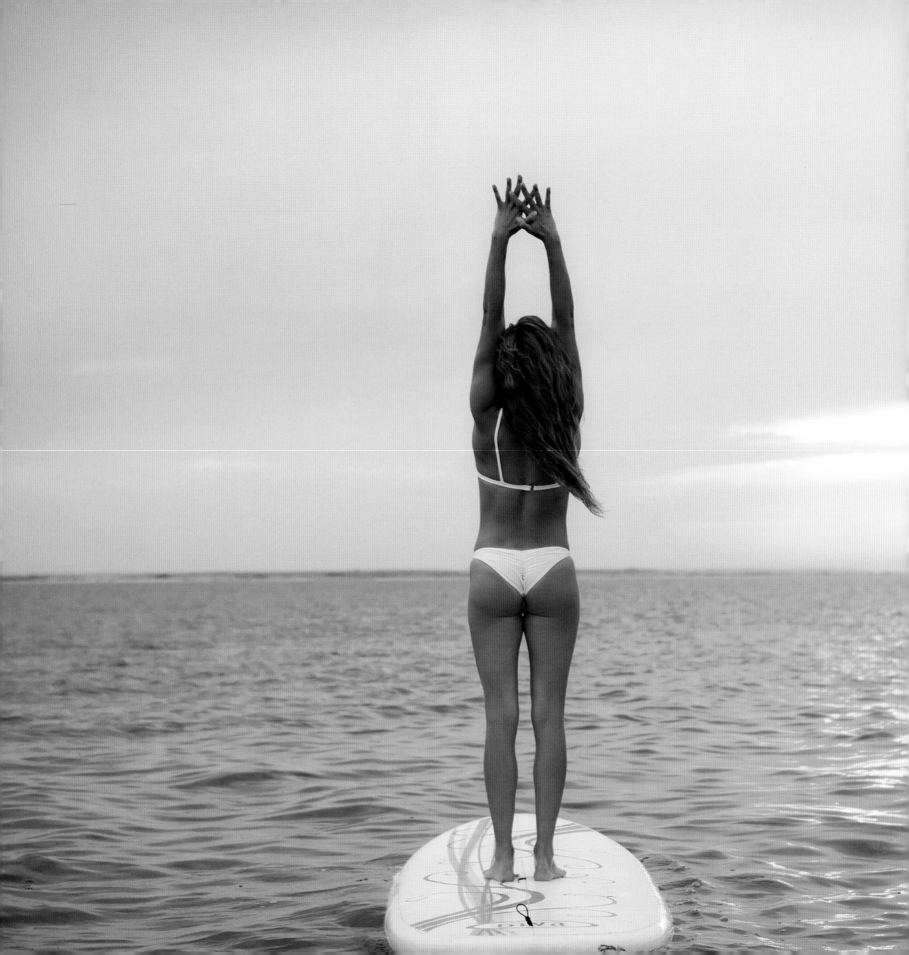

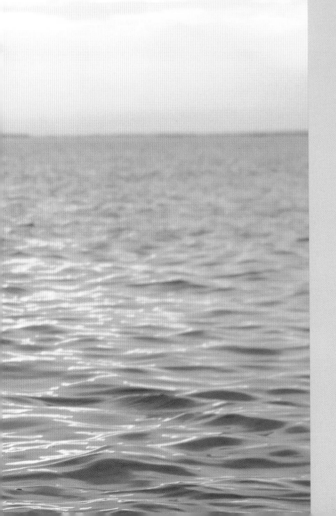

Look Up

The warm and sleepy bay of Three Mile Harbor is where I hold Paddle Diva classes during the summer. It is a serene bay, and the water is so shallow you can see the bottom. As you go deeper, the color of the water darkens to a deep blue-green that always reflects the sun with the luster of a blanket threaded with diamonds. The gentle breeze from the southwest keeps you warm and pulls you closer to the water's edge, welcoming you to dip your toes in.

Before we set off on a paddle, I remind my students where to focus their eyes. When students first stand up from a kneeling position on their boards, they either look down at the board or at the water, both of which are in motion. Focusing down will make you unsteady. We teach them immediately to simply look up at the horizon, where they want to be heading.

"While we are all kneeling on the board," I tell them, "I'll pick a still point on the horizon for you to use as a beacon to guide you through the first five minutes of the paddle. When you get to a standing position, focus on this point

1

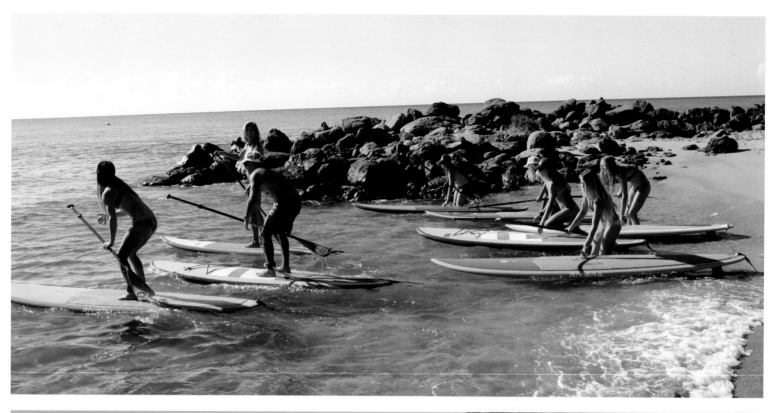

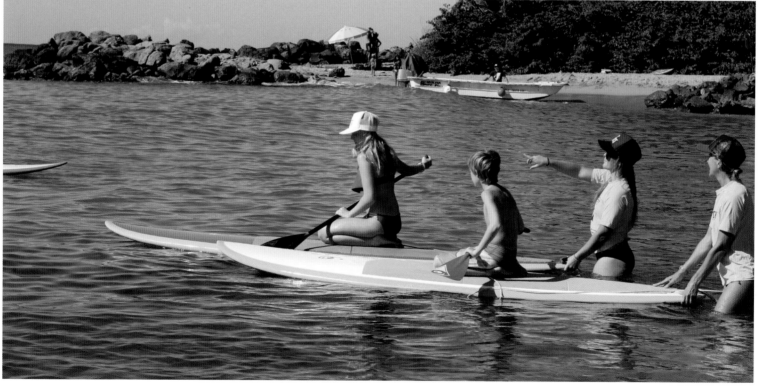

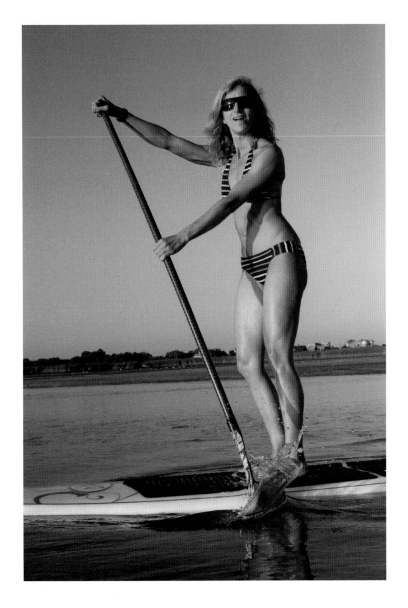

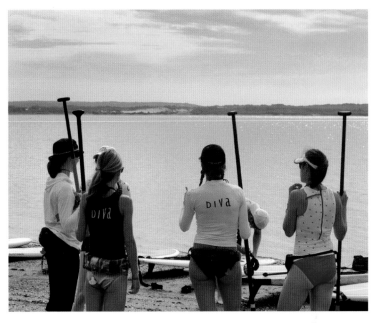

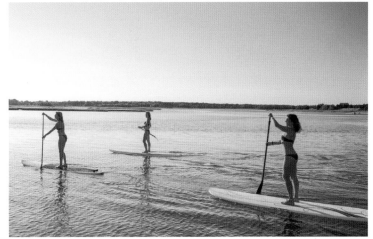

and paddle towards it. Don't look down at your board or the water. If you look down, the movement of the water will make you disoriented, and you may fall off the board and into the water. Instead, look up and focus on where you want to go."

Years ago, a student of mine was unable to take her eyes off the water and the front of her board as she attempted to stand up and start paddling. Of course, Iris immediately lost her balance and flopped into the bay. I reminded her that we don't look down when we walk because we instinctively understand that we'll bump into things and it will make it impossible for us to know which way to go. If they do take a plunge, I like to talk to my students while we are both floating in the ocean. It's soothing and helps them to relax and see that it's just water. After scooching back onto her board and into a

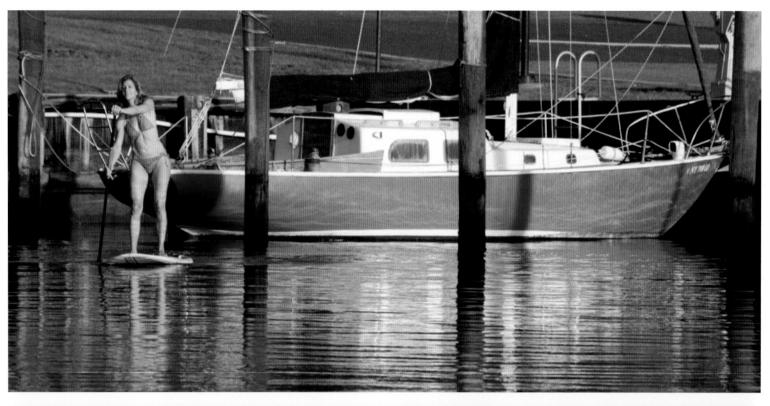

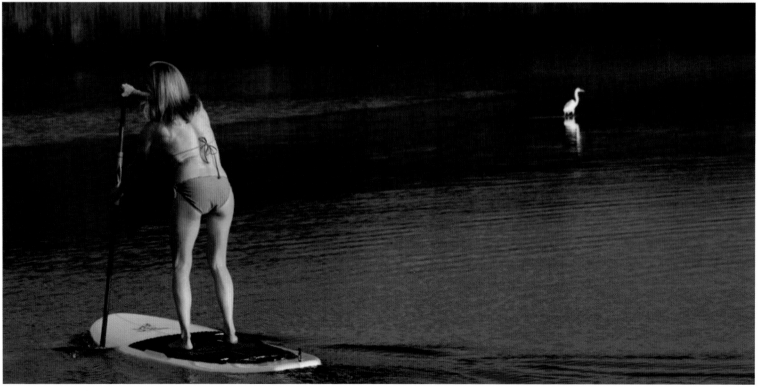

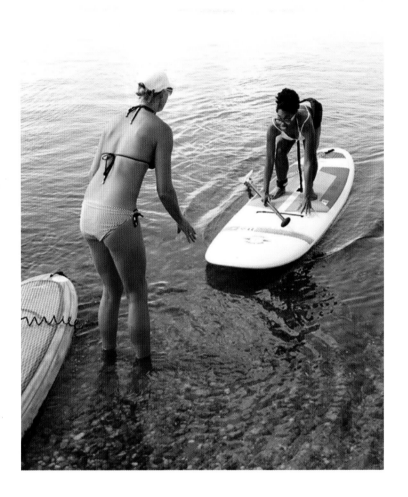

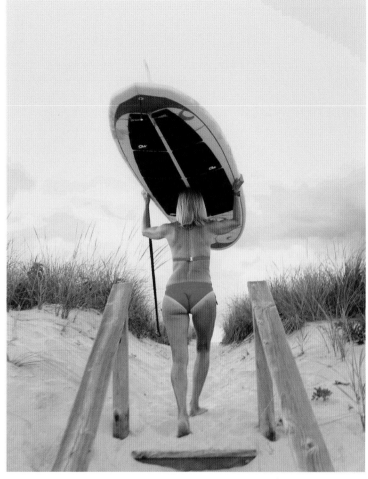

kneeling position, Iris reached her hand out to me and said, "I know, I have to look at the horizon. Saying it out loud will make me do it this time." She rose to her feet and identified her spot on the horizon. Quietly, she held her paddle in the palm of her left hand and the shaft in her right hand and started moving forward.

While we were gliding over the water, Iris explained to me that she had suffered in the past from vertigo. As a result, her perspective was a little off. She also told me that she had been preoccupied with worry that she would not be able to stay on the board. As we paddled along the shoreline, she relaxed and started looking where she wanted to get to on her board. We came upon mother and father swans out for a swim with their newborn cygnet, and we both steered away so as not to intrude on them. She learned that if she just looked up to where she wanted to go, she would be able to maintain her balance and stay on the board! Looking up opens your chest and straightens your spine, allowing you to get the most amount of air into your lungs. Iris was able to paddle the full hour, laughing and enjoying the sights of the bay. She learned that sometimes it's enough just to look up and head where you want to go!

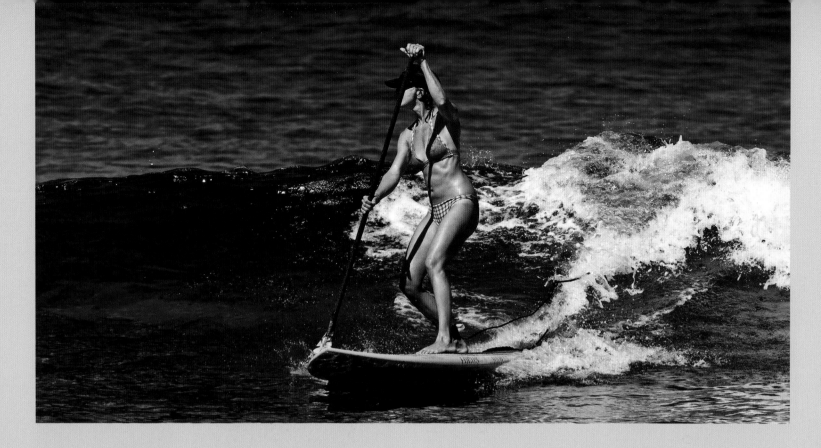

In the Moment

By Cristina Cuomo (founder and editor, *The Purist*)

I grew up in New York City and Southampton and learned to swim in the ocean. I am drawn to the sea and even took up surfing to stay connected in a deeper, more meaningful way. The mere act of surfing clears my mind as I focus on the task before me, which has enabled it to open up to greater possibilities. After all, we are made of the same property—salt water—which literally super-charges the brain by sending electrical signals that cause a heart to beat and a brain to think. The exhilarating pop-up moment after watching the wave over your shoulder that you've paddled into reminds me that, as in life, sometimes you have to look back in order to better prepare for what's in front of you.

I started thinking about my wellness brand, PURIST, when I was sitting on my surfboard in Costa Rica feeling total happiness in that moment and wondering how I could take that feeling beyond the board and share it with others. Besides bringing my children surfing with me, I was thinking about their future as a whole and how I can do my part to make it

better. As a longtime magazine editor and journalist, I realized my role—to be a catalyst for positive thoughts and actions. Thwarting bad habits in favor of healthy ones is the hardest thing to do, but through repetition and education, I found solutions to problems, not just in nutrition but in mindfulness, in physical movement, and in the home environment. I wanted to share my findings and instill this same positivity and hope in the readers of the content platform I created, PURIST.

The psychologist Timothy Leary once wrote, "Surfers are the 'throw-aheads' of mankind...the futurists and they are leading the way to where man ultimately wants to be. The act of the ride is the epitome of 'be here now,' and the tube ride is the most acute form of that. Which is: your future is right ahead of you, the past is exploding behind you, your wake is disappearing, your footprints are washed from the sand. It's a non-productive, non-depletive act that is done purely for the value of the dance itself. And that is the destiny of man."

And what a dance it is.

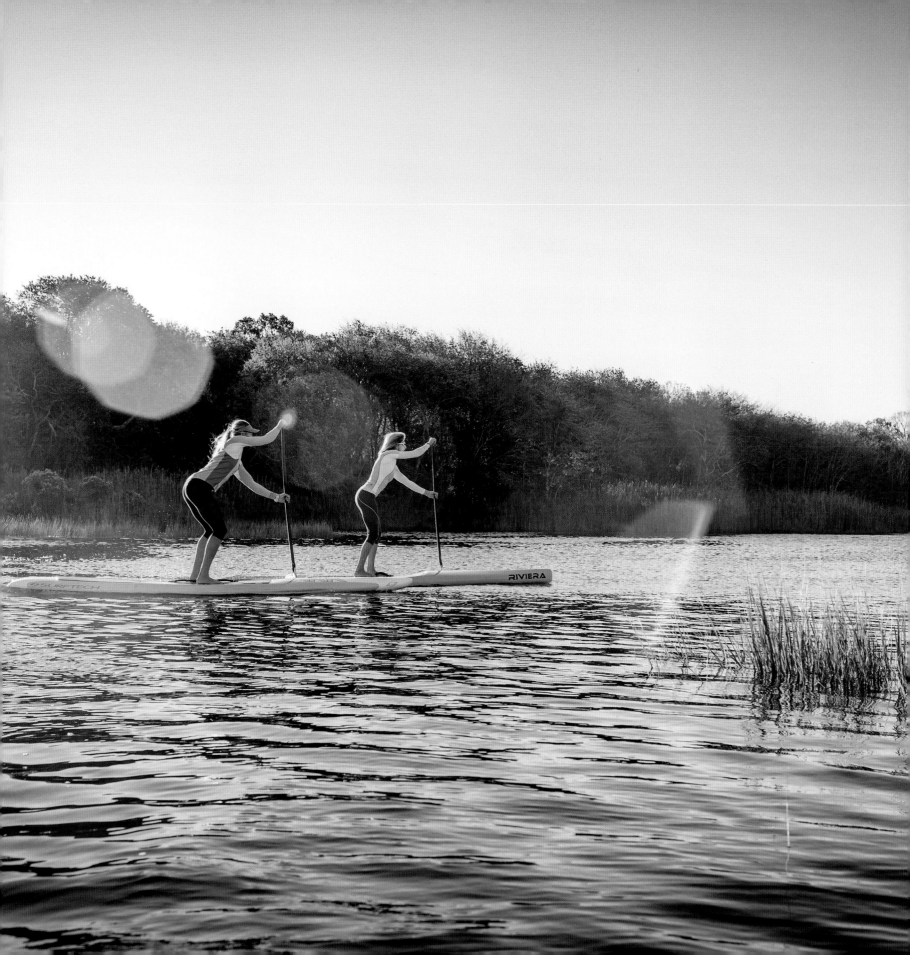

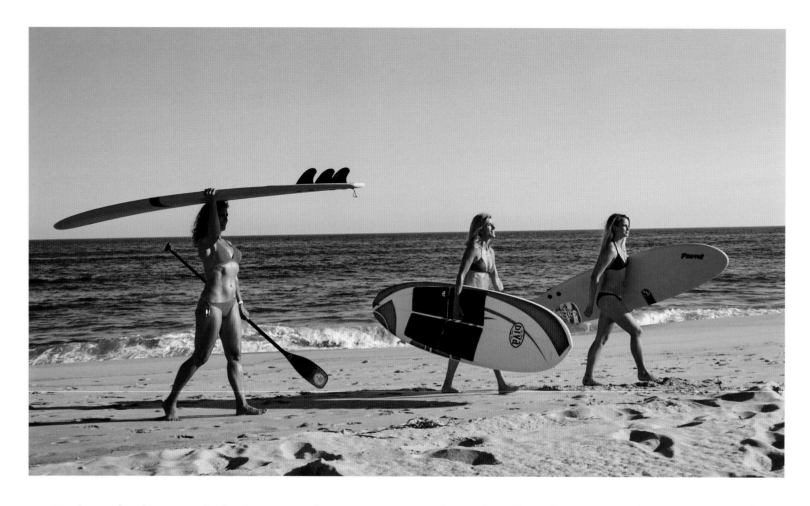

Finding a fixed spot on the horizon not only guarantees that you'll stay dry, it also allows you to self-correct. If you veer off course while you're looking up, you'll notice immediately. You want to navigate the water with two strokes on your left and then two strokes on your right. SUP requires balanced strokes; otherwise, you'll end up moving in circles. As you accumulate experience on your board, you will find a tempo, a rhythm with the water beneath you, and learn to identify when you need to increase or decrease the number of strokes on either side to keep you on your path to your destination. This Guiding Principle of balance also stresses the importance of self-correcting in life. Looking up shows you where to go, but it also allows for you to readjust your course if your destination changes, as when Iris and I paddled and came across the swan family.

It is similarly important to have a clear vision that you strive towards in your everyday life. I am a soulful person, but I am also grounded in the practical laws of the universe. I am a graduate of The Bronx High School of Science and come from a family of engineers, creatives, and scientists. I don't read horoscopes and I don't buy into psychics, but I do believe in having a vision. I know that if you have a good visualization of what you want out of life in the next hour, day, year, or decade, the rest will follow. The only way you can have a vision is if you look

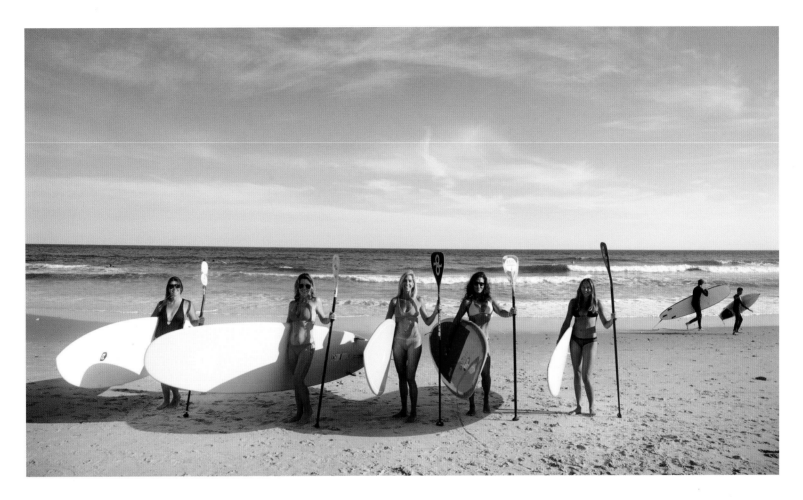

up. Look to the future and where you want to go, never where you don't want to go. It's that simple. Look up. Smile. Open your eyes wide and see what's ahead and where you want to go. Then go; go towards what you are looking at. It's yours for the taking.

One of our longtime Divas self-corrected the course of her life using this Guiding Principle. When I first met Catherine on the beach one afternoon many years ago, she was an exhausted, energy-depleted mom with two young daughters and a husband who worked five days a week in New York City and commuted out to Long Island on weekends. She felt overwhelmed with childcare during the week, she did not know what to do with the little free

time she had, it's was like she had limited visibility in the fog. She watched from a distance as I and a group of my Divas carried our boards over our heads like surfers across the warm summer sand.

We plopped the boards into the bay and took off, chatting and laughing out on the water. In that moment, looking out at the water from her beach chair, she had a vision of herself on a paddleboard, free from the stresses of her daily life. When we returned to the beach an hour later, Catherine approached me and said, "I am in. Give me your number. I love this stand-up paddling. It looks amazing. I want to be part of this too."

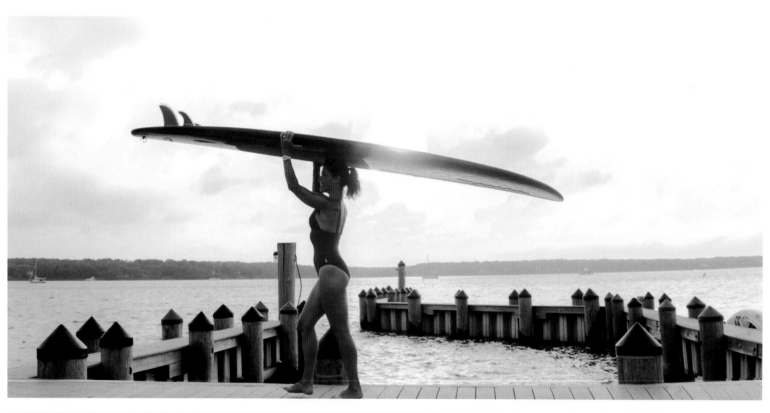

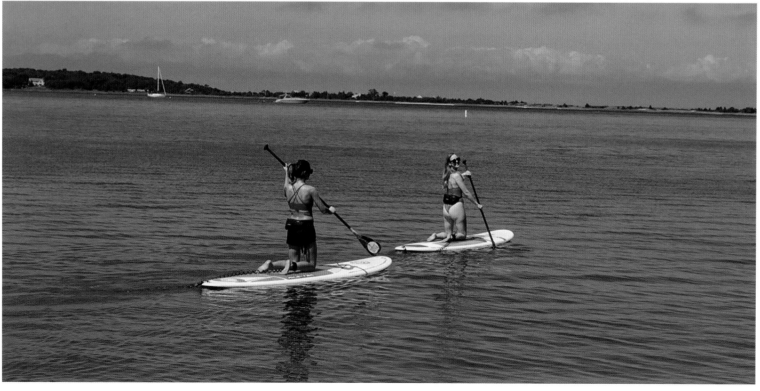

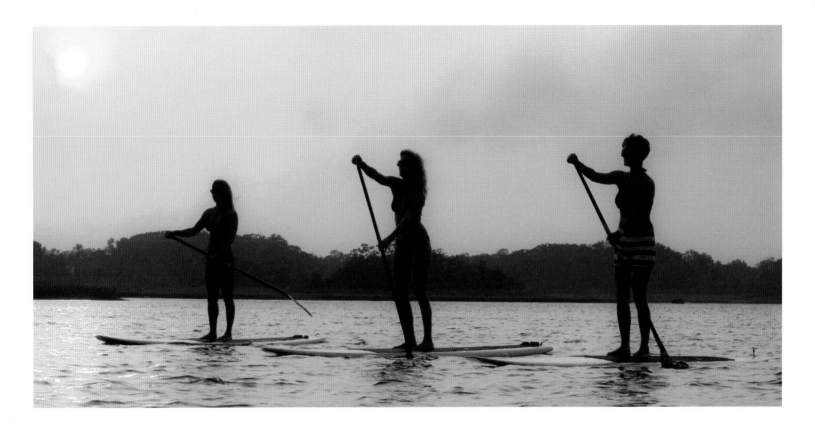

Through SUP, Catherine found that "me time" she had been craving. She was a busy mom, constantly shuttling her girls to various activities, but she always found her path back to the water. She loved it and became a Diva in no time. Catherine discovered that when she was out on the water, she was able to focus on getting in shape and be completely detached from a hectic schedule on land. For her birthday, her husband bought her a board, and she met up with us for paddling adventures. She honed her SUP skills, which gave her great confidence that summer, and loved having time to chat with the others in our group. Over time, she trimmed her figure and went back to the city ready for the autumn feeling fit and happy. Becoming a Diva and being one with the water while paddling gave Catherine a wonderful sense of herself and what she could accomplish by looking ahead and paddling toward it!

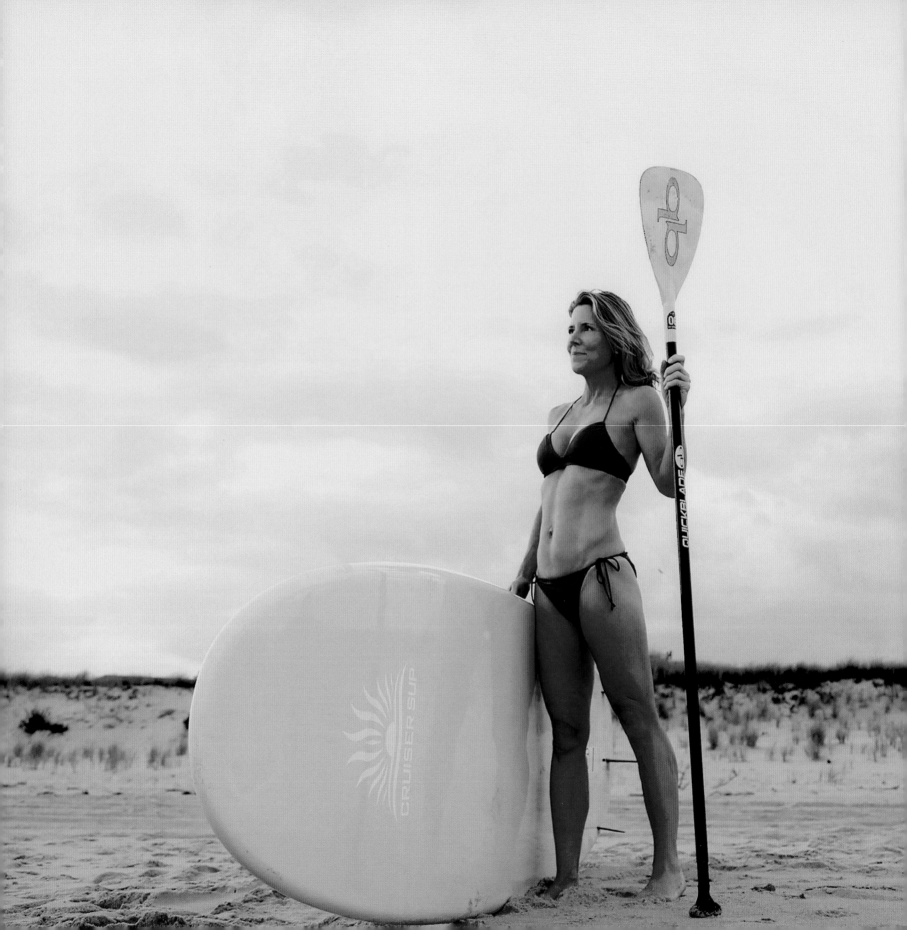

Believe in Your Strength

"SUP is one of the most inclusive sports because anyone who can walk can do it," I say countless times to my students who are feeling anxious about heading out on the calm Caribbean sea at Maria's Beach in Rincon, Puerto Rico. My classroom is under the shade of palm trees, cooled by the gentle tropical breeze and we look out to sea as I continued to teach. "We use our strength to move through the water, putting the blade in and pulling it alongside the board. That's how you glide forward over the water—powering your motion through your own strength."

So many people show up for a lesson walking and talking, then tell me they "can't" SUP. They tell me about their bad backs, their knees, their lack of sleep…in all honesty we all have some sort of bodily injury or pain that can

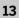

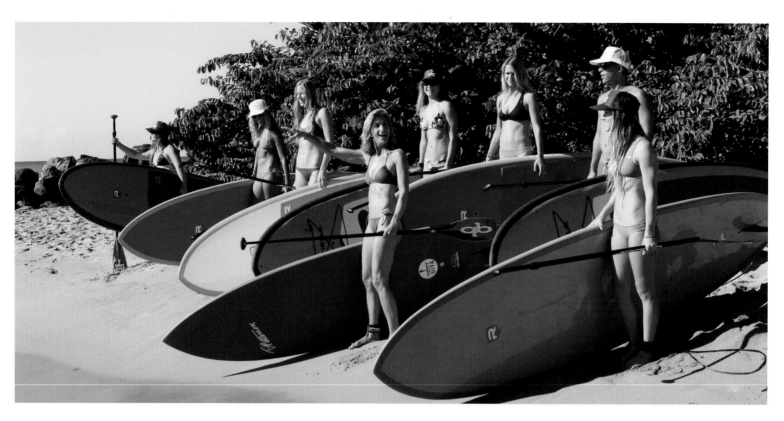

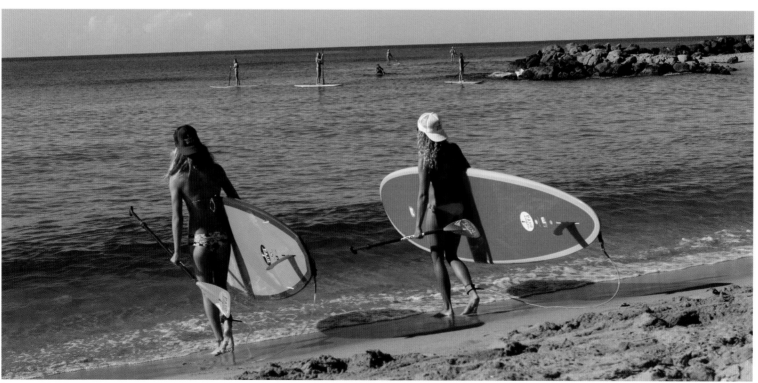

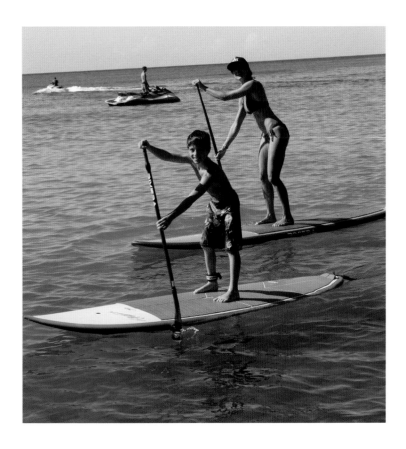

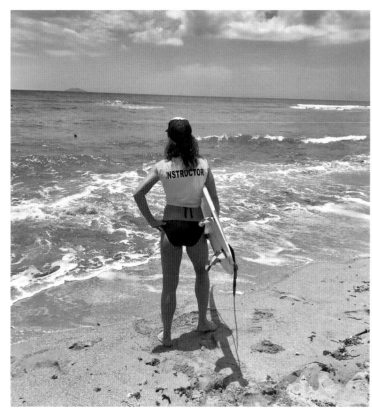

plague us from time to time. When my students show up and try to use this as a potential reason for me to bench them, unless it's truly something that precludes them from getting on the water, it's my job to educate them and flip their mindset around. There is always a solution for every problem.

One balmy Caribbean afternoon, after my morning classes were all done, a tall, athletic-looking man strode into the Paddle Diva center at Rincon's Black Eagle Marina and asked for a lesson. As we were talking about his fitness background, he took his shoe off and said, "Good luck with this." His ankle and foot appeared to have collapsed from a decades-old football injury. He was worried that he'd be a challenge for me because he couldn't transition from kneeling to standing, and he

wasn't sure he'd be able to maintain balance on the board. He doubted his strength and athleticism. As we carried our boards, paddles, leashes, and life belts down to the clear blue sea, I changed the subject of his flattened foot and ankle to what he did for exercise. As he told me about the bike riding, the rowing, and the boxing classes he took, I assured him that he actually did have the strength to paddle; he just had to believe it.

I started him off in the water from a standing position. This takes experience to do with someone, as it requires starting by standing on the board while the instructor cues the person and holds the "tail," or back of the board, to keep it balanced. It was the best way to get him to start paddling and take his mind off the lack of strength he thought he had in his foot and ankle. It was amazing to watch him balance and brace his body and feet against each stroke. I saw the moment he realized, *Hey, I can do this. My ankles are strong enough, and my feet are holding me!* Within minutes he was cruising along.

As it inevitably does in the afternoons in Rincon, the winds gently shifted from the north to the south and the water got choppy. A fishing boat motored by, creating a small wave. With this instability, my student fell into the water and then laughed as he pulled himself back up onto his board, seamlessly moving from a kneeling position to standing upright. He had completely forgotten that he thought he'd never be able to get from kneeling to standing. Turns out, he *was* able to perform this transition. He had just never given himself the opportunity to experience his full potential and did not believe in his own strength even with injury.

SUP is about having a strong mindset and focusing on your strengths instead of dwelling on any presumed or real physical weaknesses. SUP really does feel good. It's a great way to disconnect and unwind from your everyday madness. You need only to release your negative physical story to rise up on your board and enjoy the splendor of the water.

This Guiding Principle is especially important for people who struggle with illnesses or physical conditions. It's critical that you listen to your body, but you must also trust that you have the strength to overcome. I was diagnosed with scoliosis when I was seventeen. It was too late for a brace, and I refused to ever consider surgery as a means of correction. As a result, even with my living the most active balancing lifestyle, my spine is crooked, my hips are uneven, and one rib juts out. I am always in

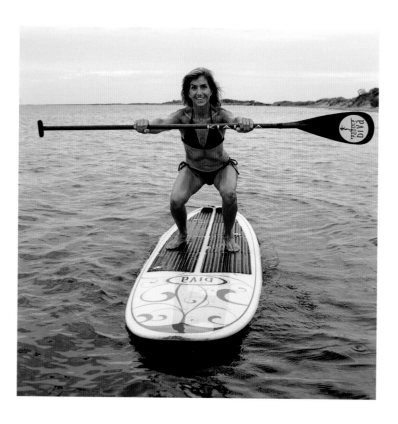

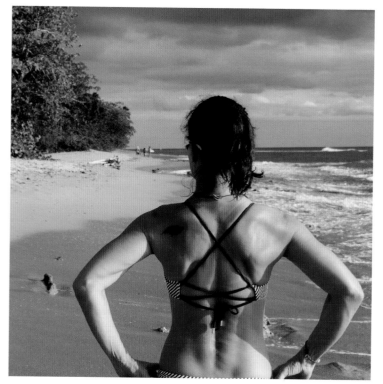

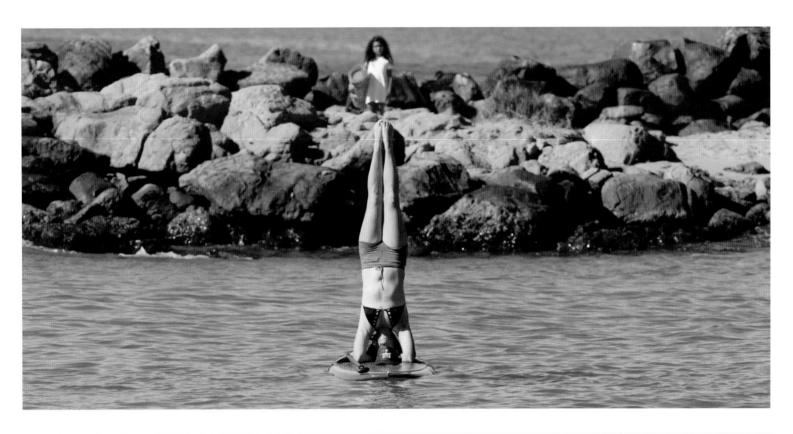

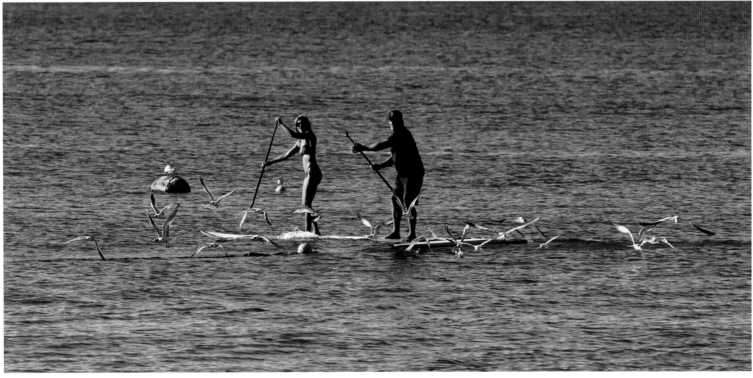

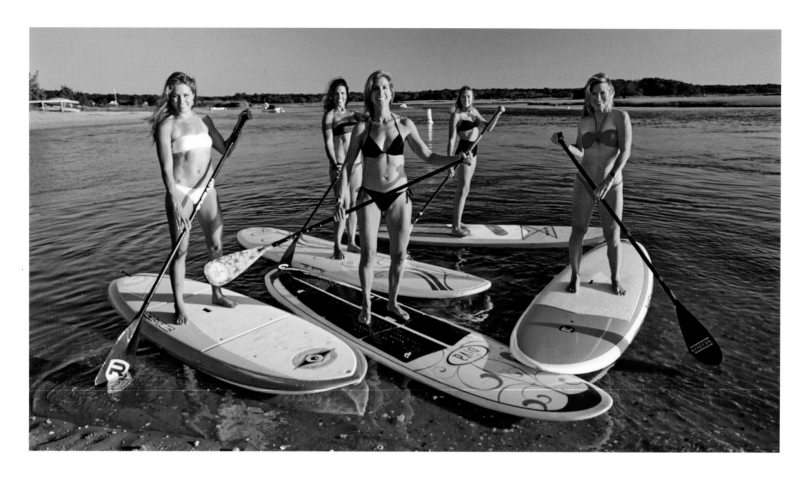

muscular pain and feel sore just about every day along my right hip and lower back. When I lean over and show my curvature, people are amazed that I am so strong, that I picked a career in wellness and watersports, and that I can lift and load a truck full of boards! I have always believed in my ability to build my core and maintain my strength to compensate for some muscles' not working as well as they should and others' working too hard. It is that belief, that I am strong and I will never give up, that keeps my body strong—and my mind follows suit.

I discovered exhale spa's barre program as my own form of rehabilitative work for my back. The spa was co-founded in 2003 by Elisabeth Halfpapp and Fred DeVito, and since then its Barre program has become the world standard in barre fitness. The results come over time, but even after one week I started to really feel the difference! I am now certified in barre through exhale's forty-hour teacher training program. I participate in classes two to three times a week, and I feel the benefits of this rehabilitative form of exercise combined with paddling. This training has also strengthened the BOGA FITMAT workouts powered by Paddle Diva, which bring a floor-based workout to an inflatable mat that floats on top of the water in a pool or calm bay.

Exhale and Paddle Diva first joined forces in 2013 when we offered an exclusive Barre + SUP class led by Elisabeth and myself. With over twenty students in each class, we were able to capture the essence of our two

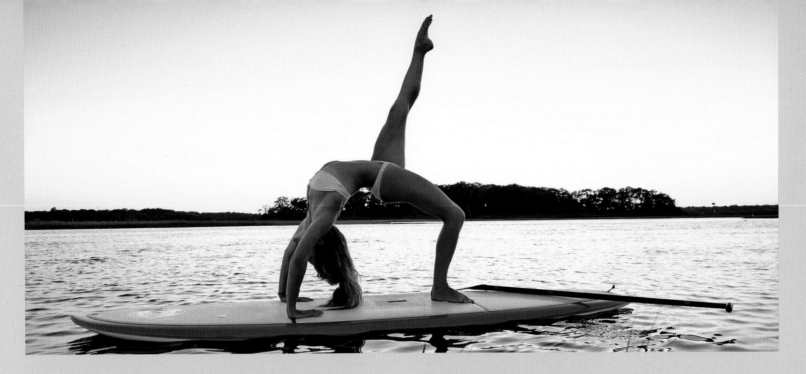

The Synergy Between SUP and Barre

By Elisabeth Halfpapp (*Co-founder of exhale and co-creator of the Barre program*)

The first time I stood up on a paddleboard, I was grateful for having a barre fitness practice. The muscles that I needed in the entire process—moving from kneeling to standing, balancing in the stance, and shifting the paddle from one side to the other—challenged my core stability, balance, and upper body and leg strength. Engaging these muscles and feeling the confidence in myself, because of my barre fitness practice, led to a very enjoyable experience on the water that gets better and better every time I go out on a board.

Barre fitness is exercise that works deeply into the layers of the muscles, providing a blend of strength, flexibility, balance, stamina, and endurance. Our priorities are based first on getting into proper position with thoughtful body alignment, then they focus on increasing reps. These are exercises that require the same focus and concentration as when you are standing on a board, as they are detailed in nature, which means they work super fast to give you results! They are highly intense exercises, but at the same time extremely safe and effective. We use positions based on dance training and sports conditioning that start with an exercise setup and proceed through a progression to challenge you in a very consistent way.

When we talk about "core strength" in a barre class, we are teaching students how to activate their main core stabilizer, the transversus abdominis. This is the deepest abdominal muscle in the body, with the primary action of compression or "pulling in." As it relates to SUP, when you pull your abdominals in, you stabilize the pelvic girdle and lower-back region, enabling you to pull the paddle through the water, switching from side to side with the greatest efficiency and support. The power achieved with the stroke is directly related to your ability to create a solid foundation from which to pull the paddle. This makes the activity more efficient, requiring less energy and work so that you can paddle for longer periods of time without fatigue.

After just a few barre classes, you will see rapid improvement and you will be doing things in class that you may never have thought were possible! This will translate to an activity like SUP, and after a short time on the water you will begin to believe in your strength and enjoy an activity that will bring you years of pleasure, combining fitness, sport, and hobby out on the water!

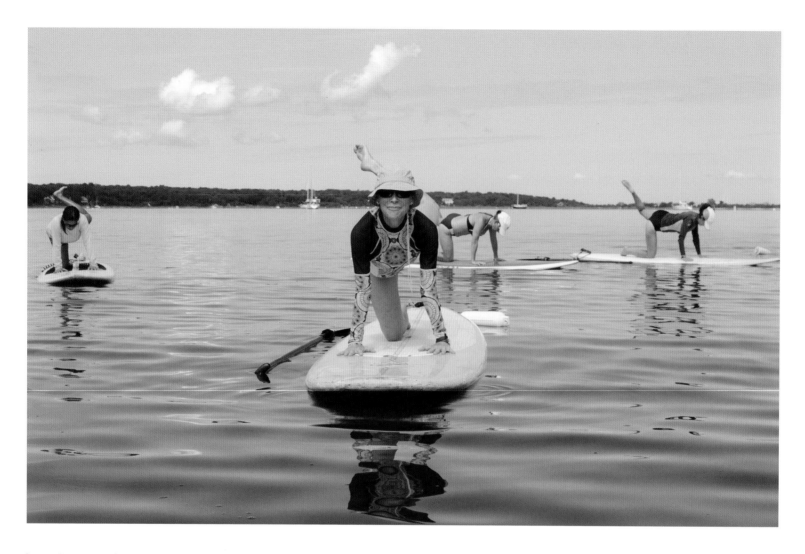

brands and offer something unique to the Hamptons crowd in the summers. Now, as I move forward as a barre-certified teacher through exhale, we will continue to explore ways to merge land and sea into one strengthening experience that helps students discover the "I can" and "I will" that are the key messages of both of our businesses!

We sometimes underestimate our own strength when faced with challenges on land. It's essential that we believe in our power to overcome any obstacles that may stand in our way. When learning how to SUP, we have to believe in this very same strength, access it, and use it to have the most amazing experience on the water. When students access this strength while learning to paddle, they become more confident, and they take this confidence back to land to use in their everyday lives. It's infinitely easier to step into challenges from a place of strength and confidence. Fred and Elisabeth lead with such a contagious energy, and over the past thirty-five years have worked tirelessly with so much faith in all of their students' abilities to be their best selves every day.

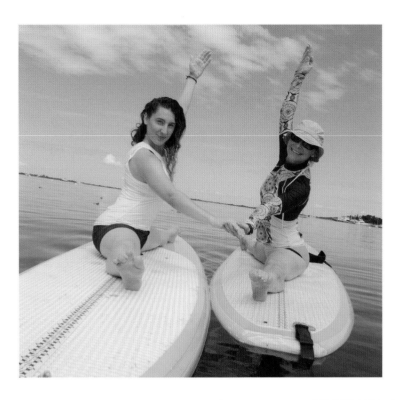

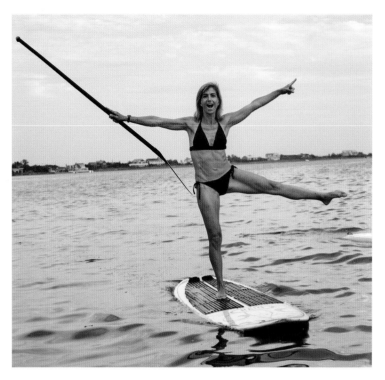

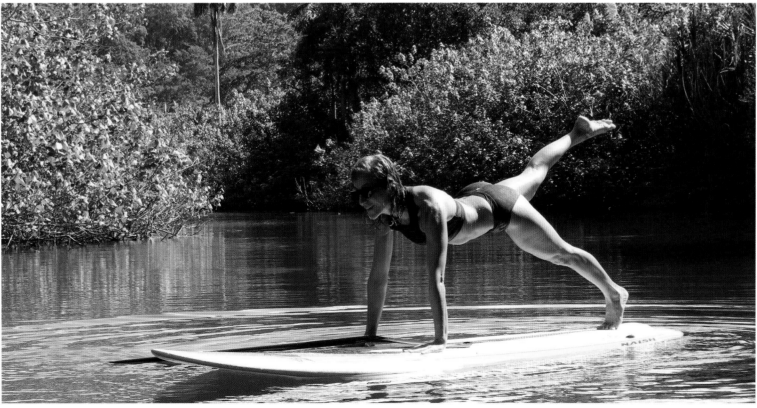

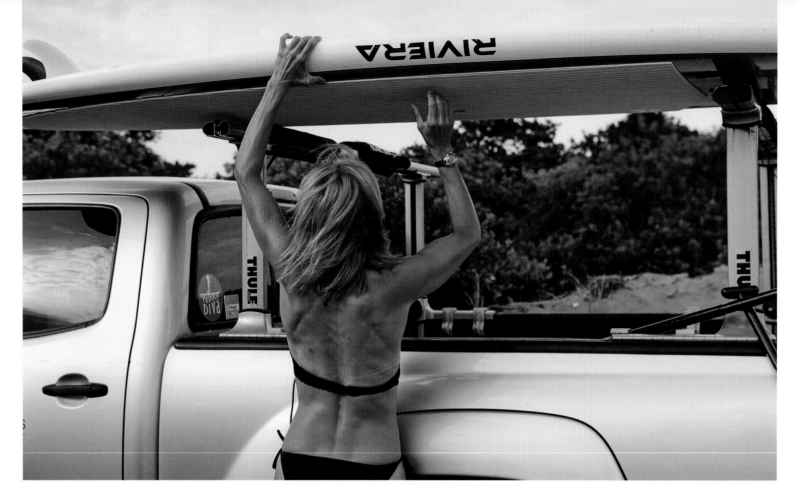

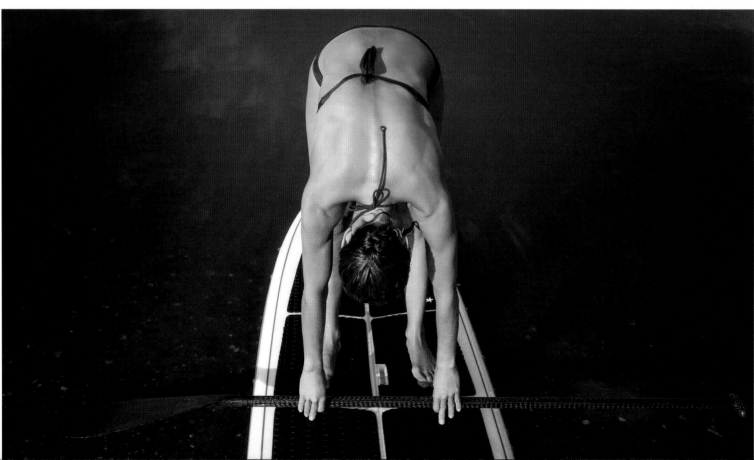

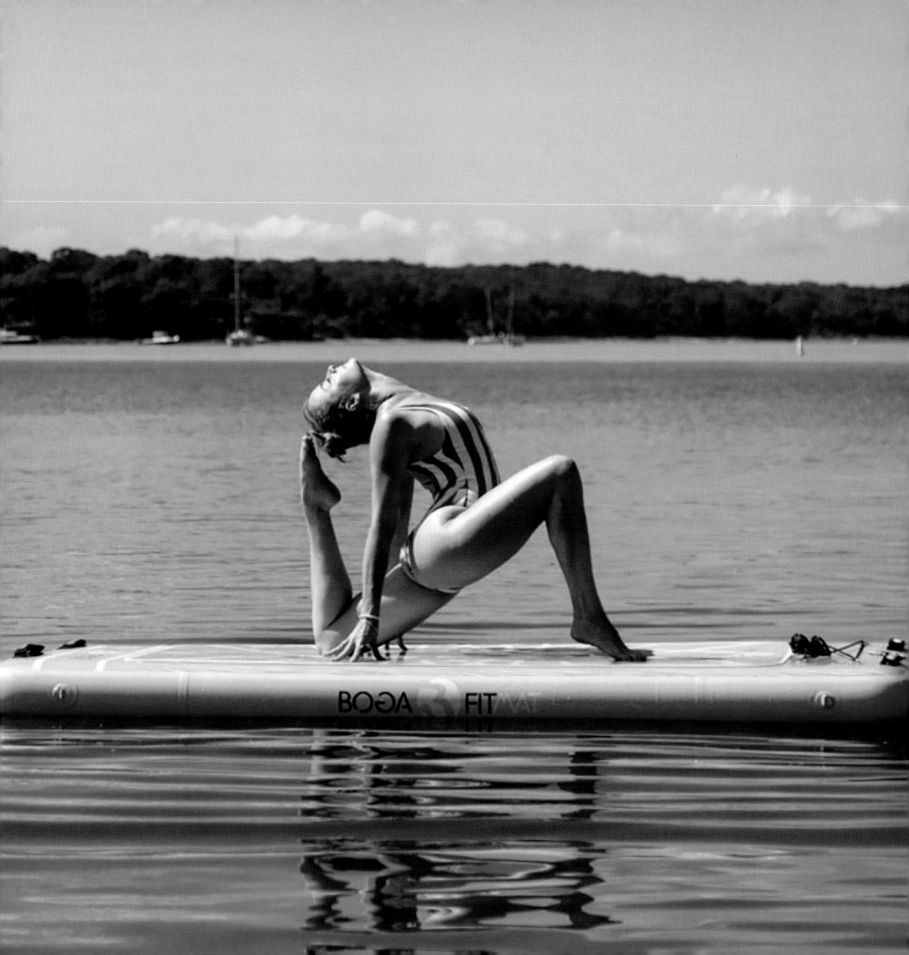

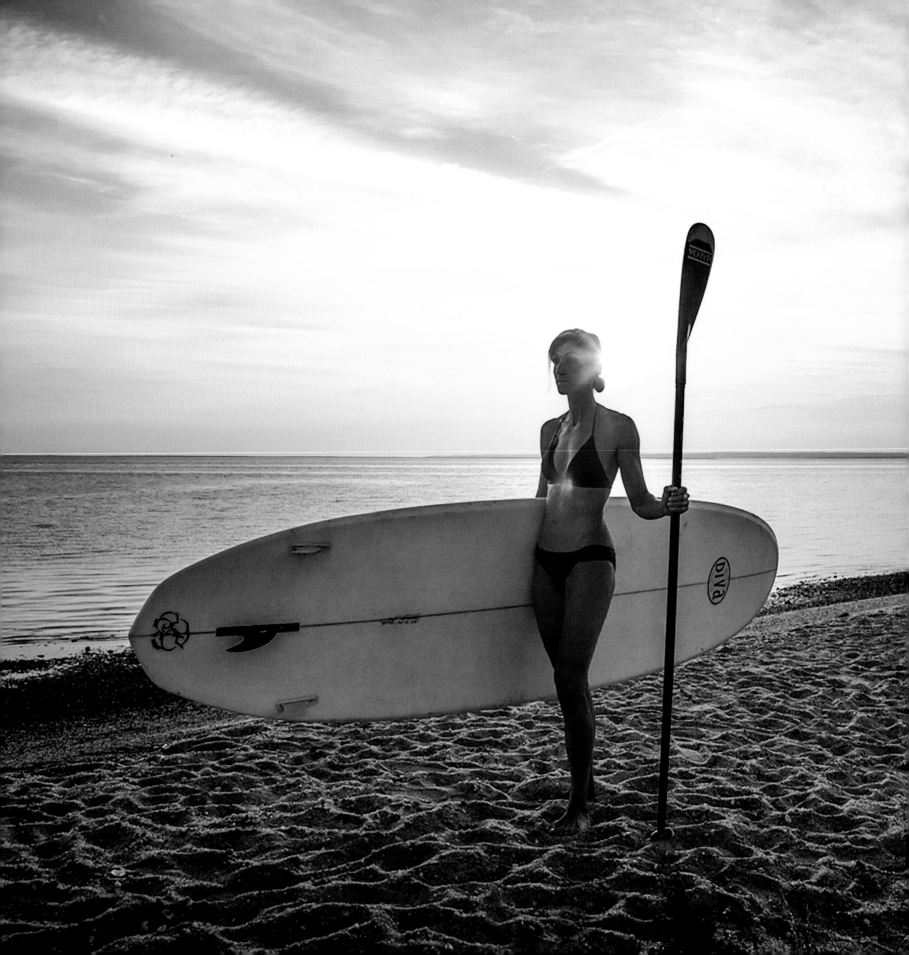

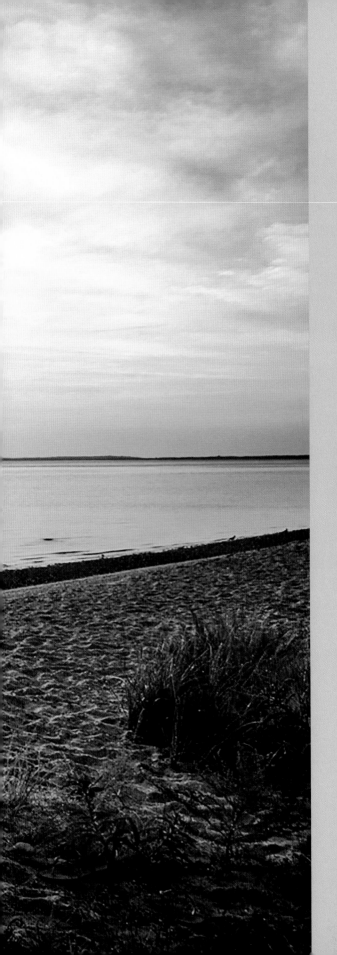

Dig Deep

Paddling *with* the wind is like having a friend's loving hand gently pressing into your back, softly steering you towards your destination. The water splashes up and keeps your feet cool. The rays of sun warm your skin. With the wind at your back, your muscles relax as you cruise even faster over the bay. I call it "flying downwind" because that's what it feels like! Paddling *against* the wind is an entirely different SUP experience. Your muscles will burn more, you may fatigue faster, you'll have to keep the front of your board facing into the wind, and you may find that it's hard to gain mileage. Although paddling against the wind is harder and more physically challenging, once you dig deep and access your strength, you will also find satisfaction in this more strenuous experience.

This same Guiding Principle shows up in our lives whenever we are faced with adversity. Whether you are dealing with an illness or the loss of a job or loved one, when life pushes you to a new limit, you must dig deep within

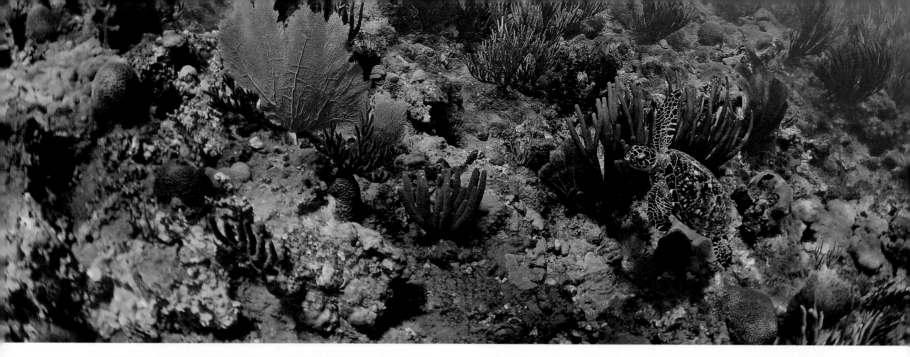

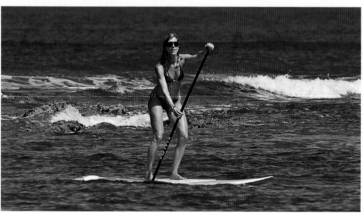
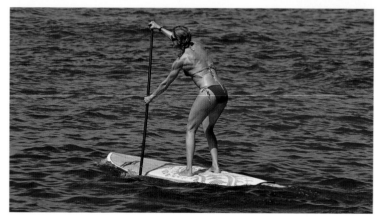

yourself and push back to keep moving forward. Helen, a former student turned instructor, has been training with me for years. She is a Diva who knows how to access her inner strength and dig deep no matter the winds, surf chop, or seas. Despite being an elite athlete, Helen struggled for a long time with an irrational fear of white water, which often occurs even in the sleepiest bays when waves are churned up on windier days. But she learned how to dig deep to get up and over those breaking waves.

It was a warm and sunny day at Maria's Beach in Rincon, Puerto Rico. Helen and I had set out on a group paddle from Maria's to Tres Palmas Marine Reserve, a

fish and reef sanctuary where we would snorkel while still attached to the boards by our leashes. Tres Palmas is home to one of the largest and healthiest elkhorn coral colonies left in the Caribbean. The ocean floor is blanketed with bright yellow antler-like formations that reach almost to the surface of the water. The reef is brimming with life. Colorful tropical fish and all sorts of fluorescent soft corals whimsically dance in the current as the gentle swells move the water sleepily back and forth. Crabs and lobsters peek out from small caves. Turtles are a common sight as they shyly swim by on their way in from or out to the ocean's depths.

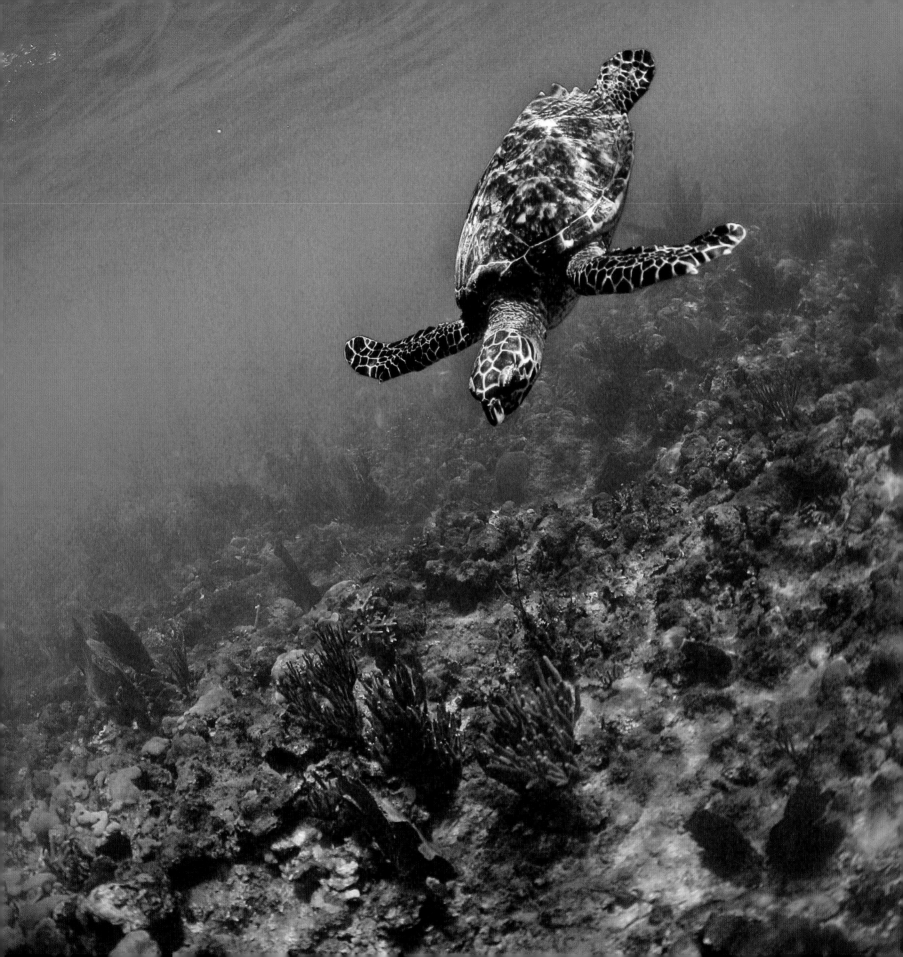

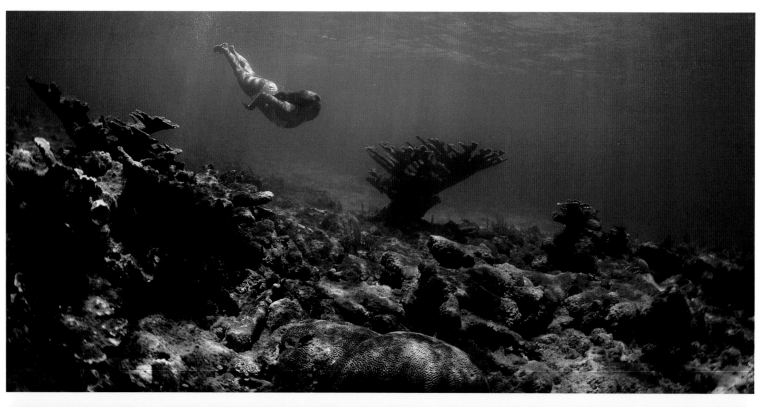

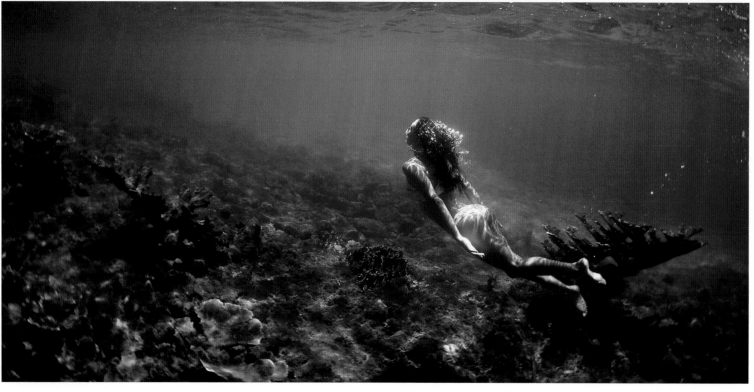

Due to high winds that day, in order to reach the underwater preserve, about thirty minutes away, we would have to paddle into the wind to cross over small, gently breaking waves. As the rest of the group made their way over the break, I looked over at Helen. Her face was frozen at the sight of the white water, and she had stopped paddling. I called her name and we locked eyes. I said, "Helen, they say the ocean always wins, but don't give in because today *you* are going to win. Now, look out to the reef and paddle like you mean it. Dig deep and paddle, paddle, paddle!" She nodded, clenched her teeth, and dug her paddle deep into the water. Instantly, her board lifted up and gently glided over the white water.

Within six quick, strong strokes she had made it out to the calm, deep blue waters beyond the breaking waves. She and I looked at each other again, and a smile spread across her face. She had conquered her fear and knew she could do anything from that point on. Since that day, Helen has become one of our top recreational paddlers, winning many local races and placing first at the Great Peconic Race around Shelter Island, New York, in 2018. She is an instigator and encourages so many to learn to SUP and join the Paddle Diva tribe. Helen is also a lighting designer and builds custom lights. She has set business goals for herself and achieves them each time. She knows what it means to dig deep.

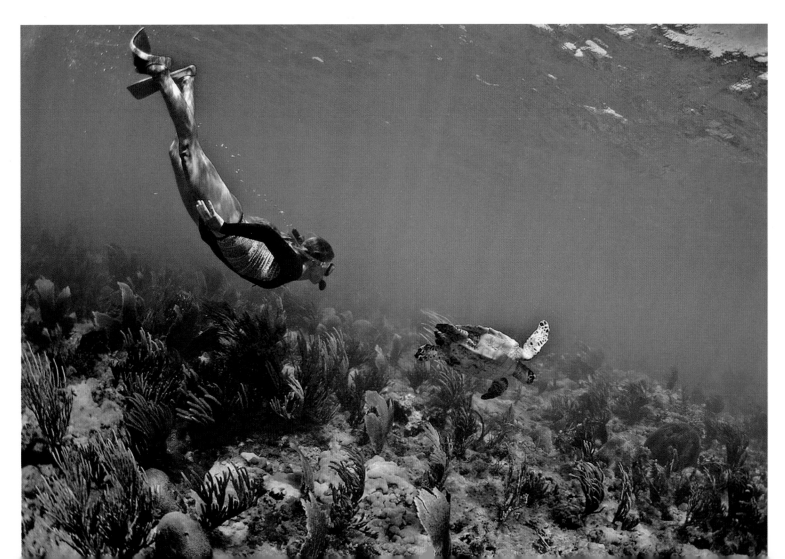

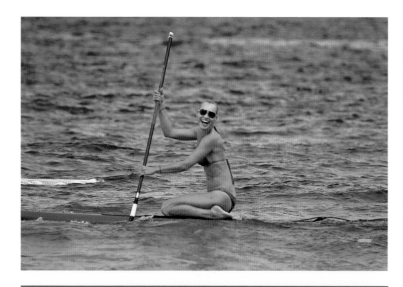

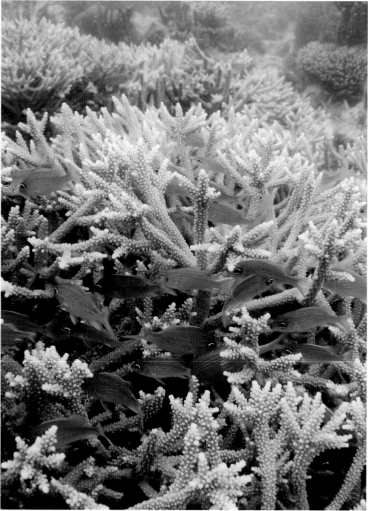

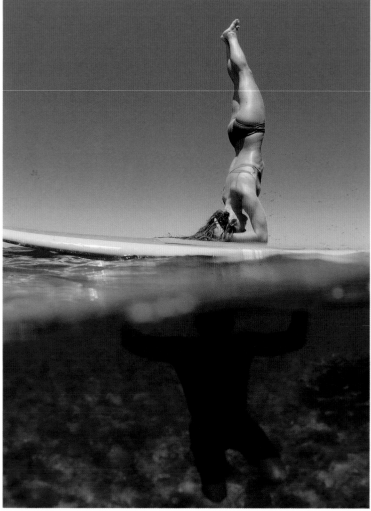

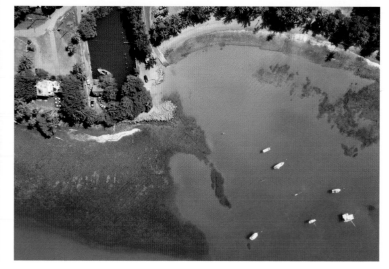

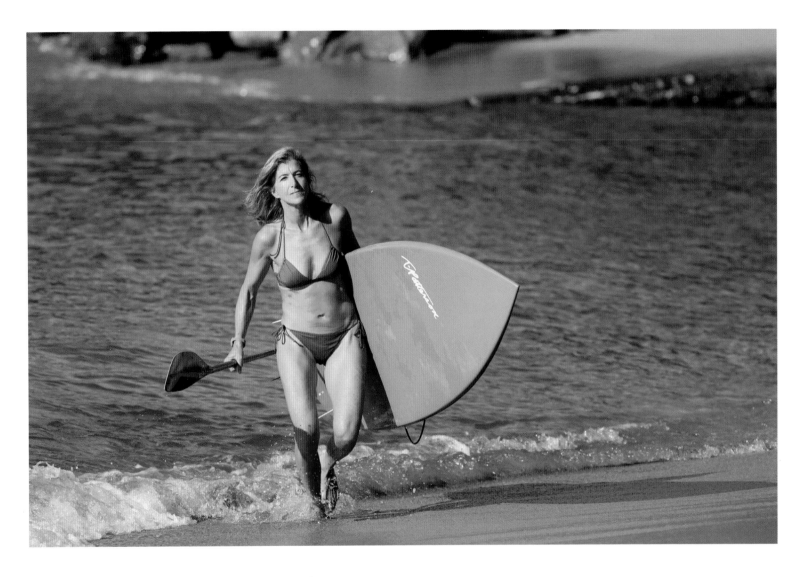

Puerto Rico has had its own experience with digging deep. In 2017, Hurricane Maria devastated the island, after Hurricane Irma had already given that region quite a blow. As a homeowner in Rincon, I did not get back to the island until the power was restored five months after the storm. This island and its people demonstrated tenacity and grit to overcome and recover after such overwhelming devastation. Many lived for months with no electricity or other power but found ways to continue to clean up and improve their neighborhoods.

The remarkable stories of recovery and reconstruction during the storm and its aftermath share one common thread: what it means to dig deep to find the strength to survive.

In the wake of Maria's devastation, Puerto Rico was left with no power and very limited resources for months. Humanitarians and activists like Bethenny Frankel mobilized quickly to respond to the island's desperate pleas for help. Through her B Strong foundation, which she began in 2017 as an initiative to help disaster victims in Houston

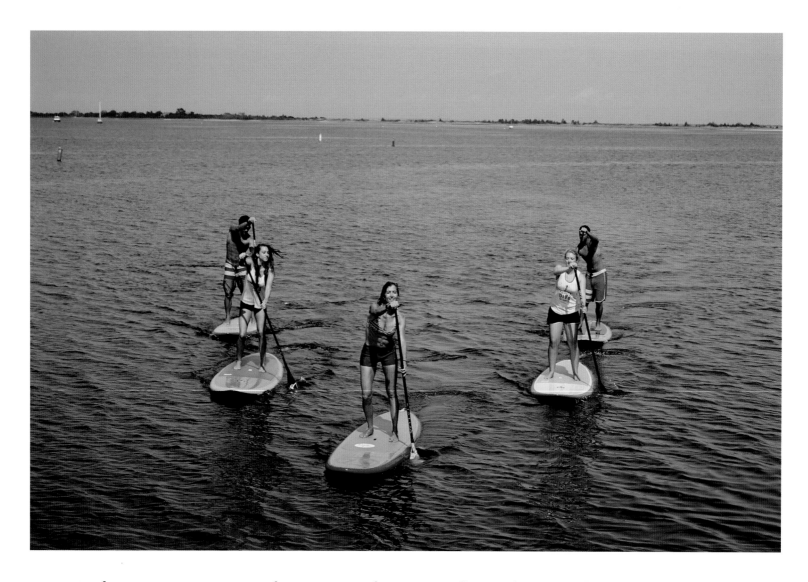

recovering from Hurricane Harvey, Bethenny organized and obtained fifty-five donated planes and filled eighty-six containers loaded with emergency aid, food, essential supplies, and gift cards that went to directly to the inhabitants of areas in the Caribbean hit hardest by the storm. She brought back elderly islanders who needed care immediately and rescued dogs, pulling ticks and fleas from their fur and finding them forever homes. Most important, she gave people a sense of hope, supported them, and let them know help was there for them.

Following that extraordinary effort, Bethenny and B Strong have teamed up with charities such as Delivering Good and Global Empowerment to help victims of natural disasters around the world. Most recently, in the fall of 2018 when hurricanes hit North Carolina and Florida's Panhandle, she was raising money, loading trucks, and going to the areas to support and inspire the victims of these disasters. Long ago, we met on a paddleboard. She was one of my first clients to design her own branded SUP board for her company, Skinnygirl. She is a celebrity

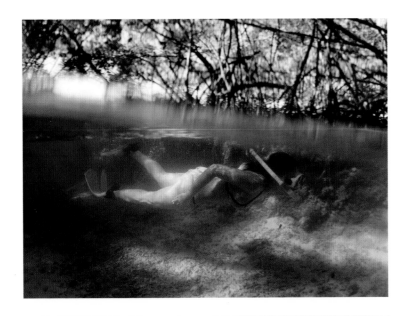

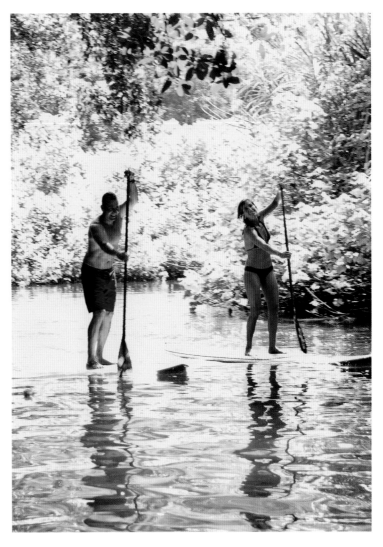

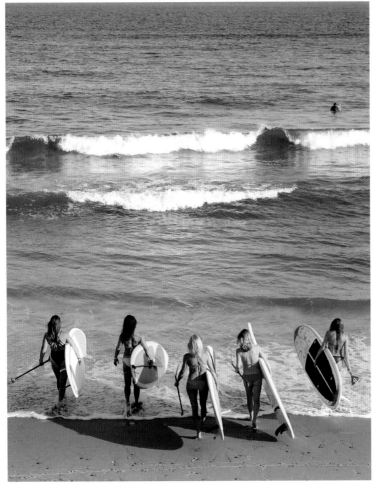

who can also paddle and has completed the entire race-course at the Paddle for Pink in 2014 and 2015. In hard winds and choppy sea conditions, Bethenny showed the crowds she is an athlete and a paddler as she crossed the finish line, arms raised in victory. Whenever she is out on the water, Bethenny paddles with such determination, strength, and grace. She is someone who knows what it means to dig deep on land, in her life, and on the water.

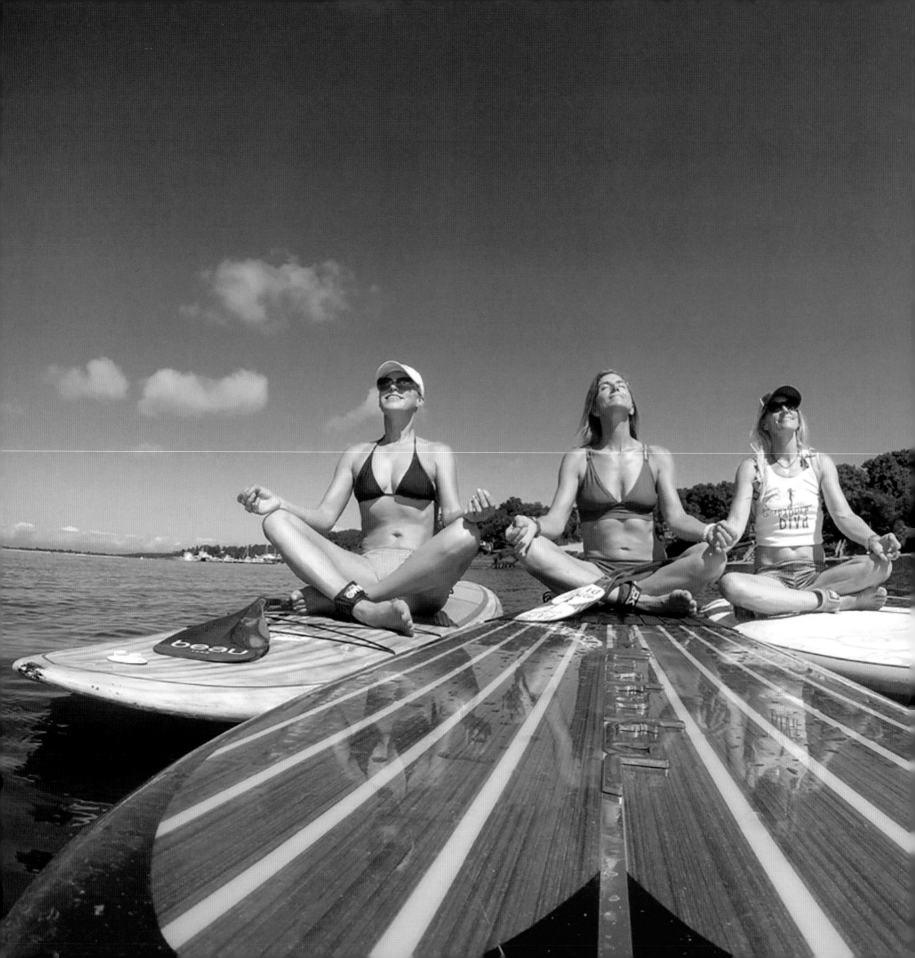

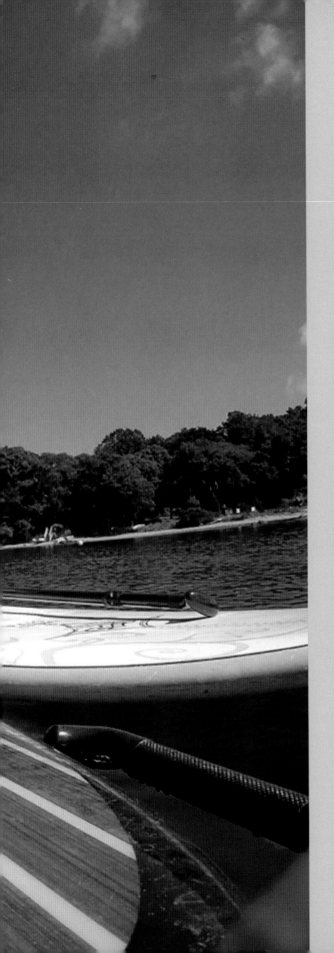

Focus on Your Core

When you tap into your core on your board, your strokes are graceful and fluid. There is a term my dear friend Jimmy Minardi uses for all of his yoga, cycling, and weight-training modalities: "effortless effort." I love this term because if you are using your core properly and paddling with the proper stroke and the right-size paddle, you can glide for longer distances and your balance is better, so you feel safer and more in control. I regularly remind my students, "If your arms hurt, you are not using your core. If your lower back is sore, you are not using your core. If your calves are burning, you are not using your core. Paddle and pull from the inside out." Then I sneak in Jimmy's words: "You want to have effortless effort, nice and easy, using your body perfectly in sync with your movement."

35

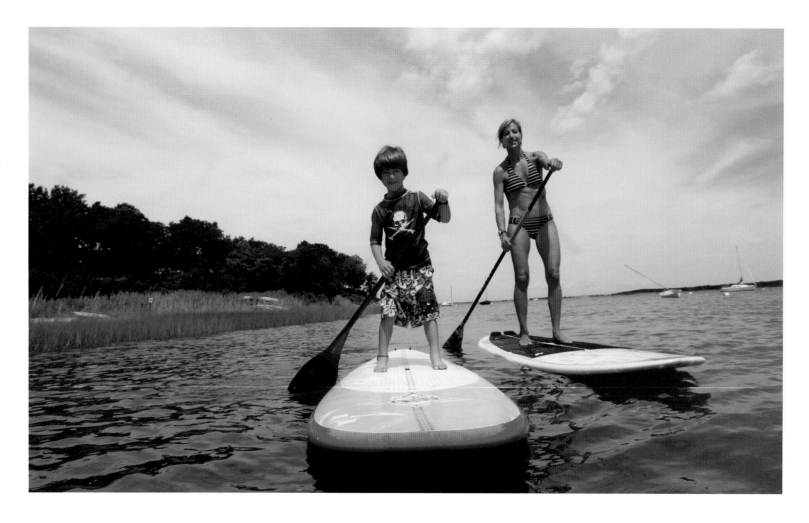

In the winter months, you can find Paddle Diva at the Boca Raton Resort & Club in Florida. It's a magical place, with its coral exteriors and Spanish style architecture. The resort has two hotels, one on the Atlantic Ocean and a second on the Intracoastal Waterway. We paddle in Lake Boca, which is a large sandbar that makes for great paddling in waters deep enough to stand. During President's Day weekend, my family was lucky enough to join me. My son James had finished playing eighteen holes of sunrise golf and was happy to be my sidekick as I worked all day. The winds from the north made the day cooler than usual but the sun was the perfect complement,

warming us up as we biked along the greens of the eighteenth hole on our way to the Marina for the Simply SUP beginner lessons at ten o'clock. James was only eleven at the time, but he's been paddling since he was about three. He's a strong paddler, and he's a natural as he uses his core and his innate athletic skills. He's a great help when I teach and he quickly sized-up the six students with paddles of the proper length. Together we launched from them from the dock, showing them how to get on the boards kneeling to start. James then showed them how to get from a kneel to stand and then how to steer the boards. One of my students from the class remarked how

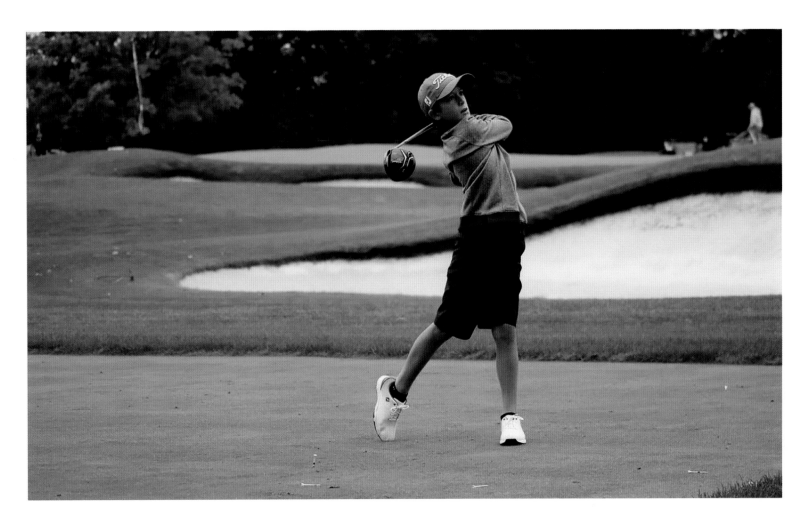

amazing it was to see such a strong kid. "It's all in his core," I explained. "Every time you drive your paddle into the water and pull back, it's like doing a crunch. The more you use your core muscles, the easier it is to paddle. Kids are the best because they have strong core strength." As we all made our way north into the wind, the students began to feel what I was saying. They used their core strength to paddle and we gently glided along the gorgeous blue green waters.

My kids are always in my core. They came from my core, and now they are my core. They are what motivates me every day to work, take care of the environment, and take care of myself. Both James and my daughter, Emma, were raised on the water—surfing, swimming, and stand-up paddling. They are both amazing paddlers, but they have picked a life on terra firma and have gravitated to land sports that they are motivated to do. My husband and I have taught them to have a strong core, or foundation, and from that they have been able to find passions of their own. Emma is a working equestrian, and James is a dedicated golfer—sports that use their core muscles and keep them very centered, much like the paddleboards they were both raised playing on from the time they could walk.

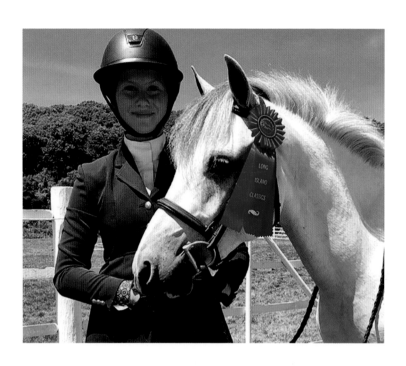

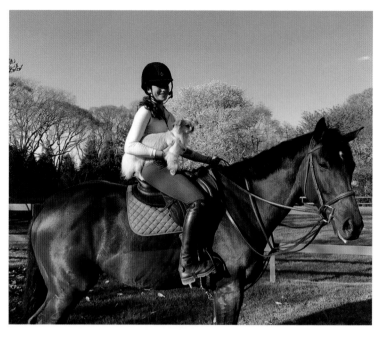

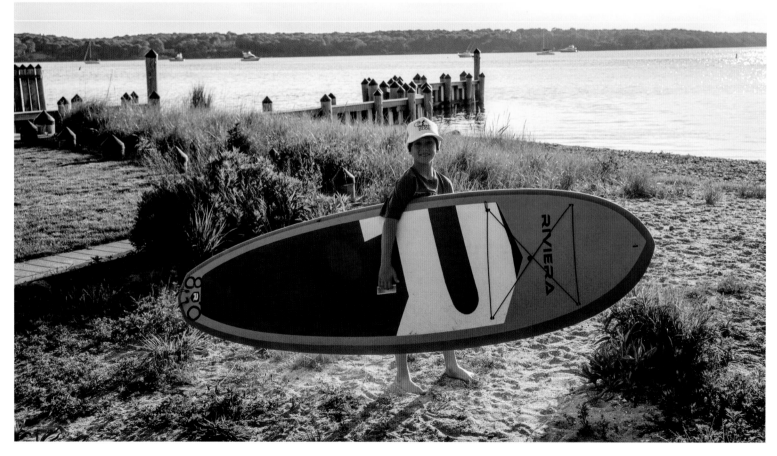

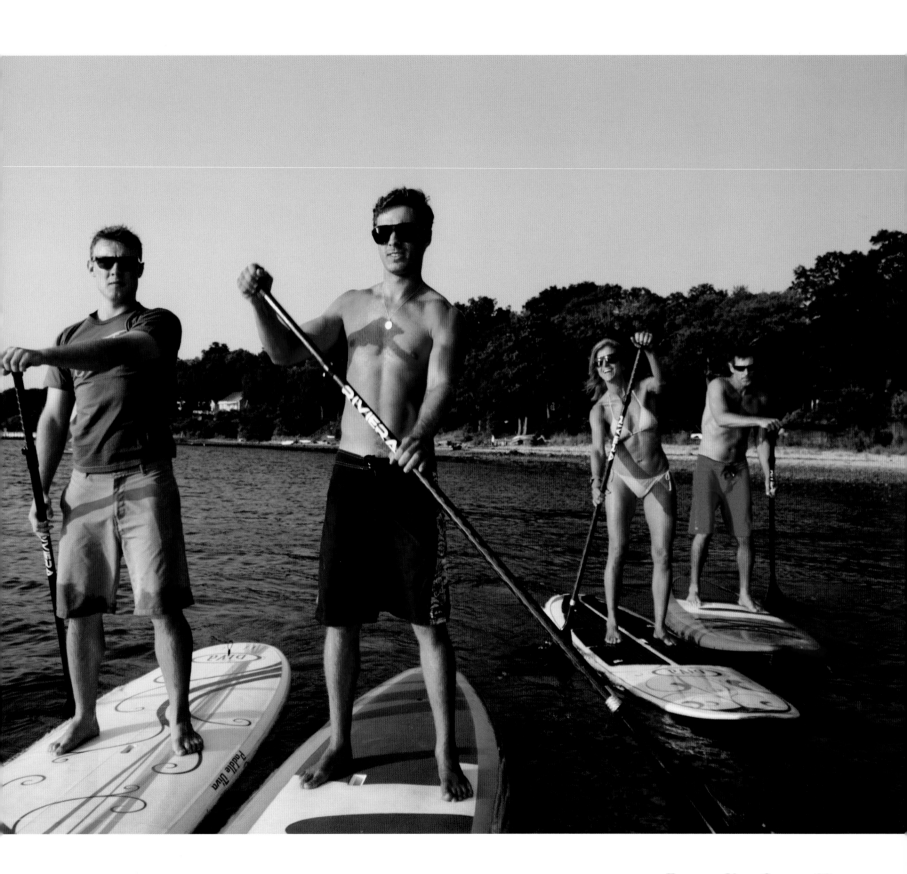

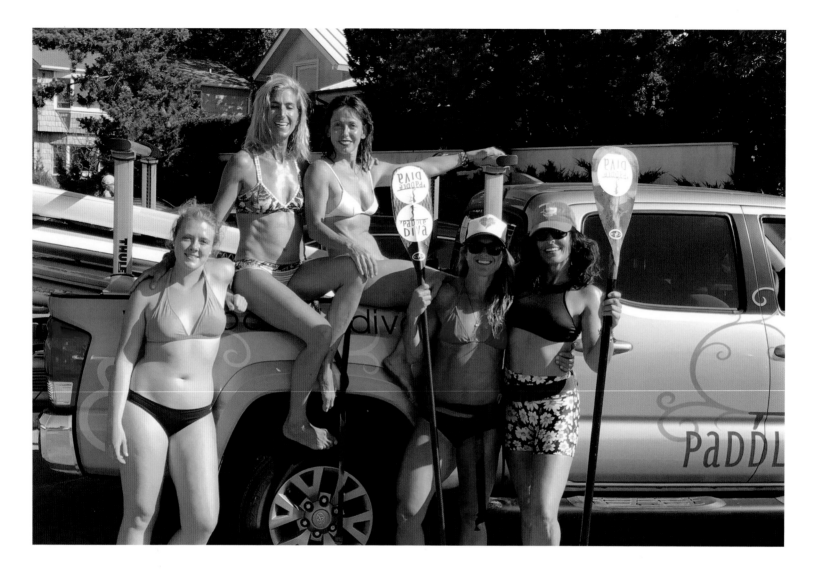

As our group paddled, the winds started to pick up and the tide began to shift creating a bit of a current that generated more resistance. Nudging them along, I showed them proper stroke technique—straight arms, driving the paddle deep into the water, slight hinge at the hip and then pull along the side of the board. As we all leaned into each stroke, with James in the front, we made our way to the sand bar and jumped into the ocean to cool off. We needed a break, to allow our muscles to relax and reset for the return trip.

Shortly after we got back up on our boards, a manatee swam alongside and we watched as he popped his head out of the water, took a breath, and then dove back down to head to the docks. Manatees tend to gather in the shade of moored boats, looking for fresh water that may be running from the docks. James pointed out how gentle the sea creature was and asked me why it had such a large scratch along its back. "Boats hit them by accident, which is why there is always a speed limit here," I explained. "At one point they almost became extinct.

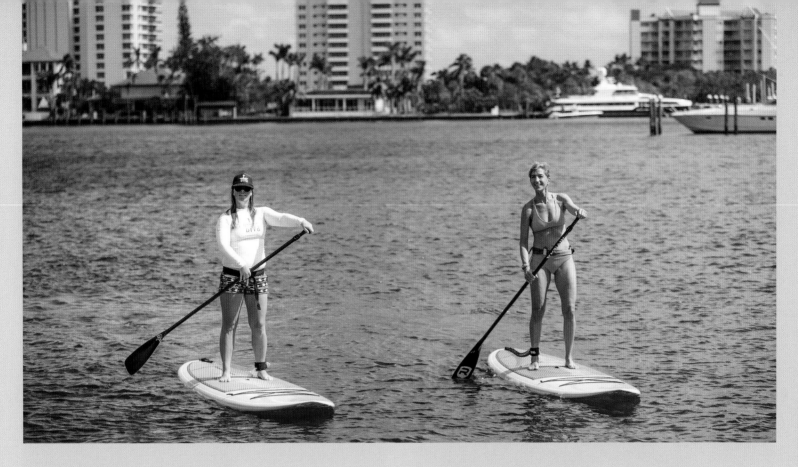

Be a Steward of the Sea

I quickly learned that I had a platform—my paddleboard—and while on it I could speak to my students about the issues surrounding our bays and waterways. While spending endless hours gliding across the bays, oceans, rivers, lakes, and ponds, you see much of humankind's impact on the environment. There are obvious signs—deflated balloons, plastic bottles, boat parts, and general pollution—but what is less apparent to the untrained eye is the various algae blooms. These are also known as "harmful algae blooms" when they start to produce toxic bacteria that poses a threat to aquatic life in the waters pervaded by these blooms.

You may hear about brown tide, red tide, rust tide, and cyanobacteria (blue-green algae). All of these have a direct impact on public health. Have I started to scare you yet? I hope not, but as a steward of the sea, I make it my business to educate my students about the threat to our precious oceans and what they can do to be a part of change. This change will occur thanks largely to the multiple non-profits that are scouring the planet in search of environmental problems and then advocating change.

As we glide along, enjoying the air, the sun, and the gentle breezes from the winds, I like to let my students know four things they can do, today, to be part of the solution:

1. **Reduce, reuse, and recycle.** This is such a common set of three words we hear often, we see on all our garbage cans, and we read about in the news. Keeping pollution out of our waters will have a direct impact on the overall health of the planet.
2. **Stop fertilizing your lawn.**
3. **Maintain or upgrade your septic system** to prevent wastewater from leaking and seeping into waters nearby.

My last point that I always make is that we all need to share this information with someone, and together we can all become advocates for the oceans.

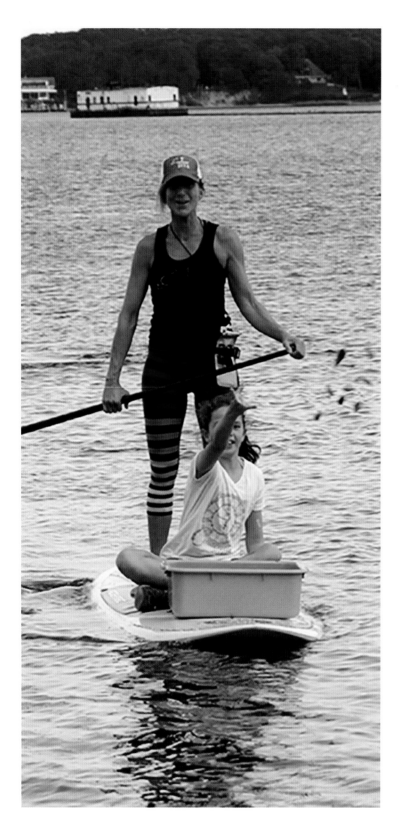

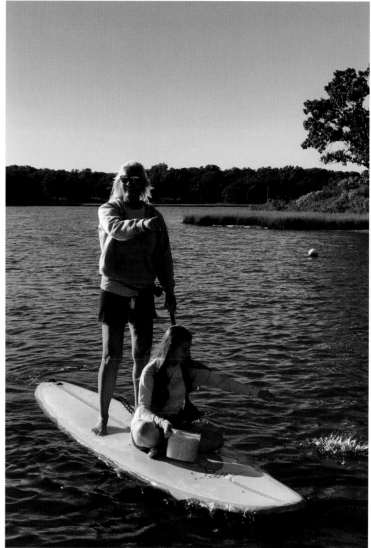

They can also be sickened by the red tides which come and go in the heat of the summer months." I went on to explain to the class that humans have created this problem through overdevelopment and pesticide use, but that it's not too late to reverse the harm we've done. I like to share my views on environmental awareness and how we can help, planting "seeds of hope" in each student and giving them something to do as a take away at each location.

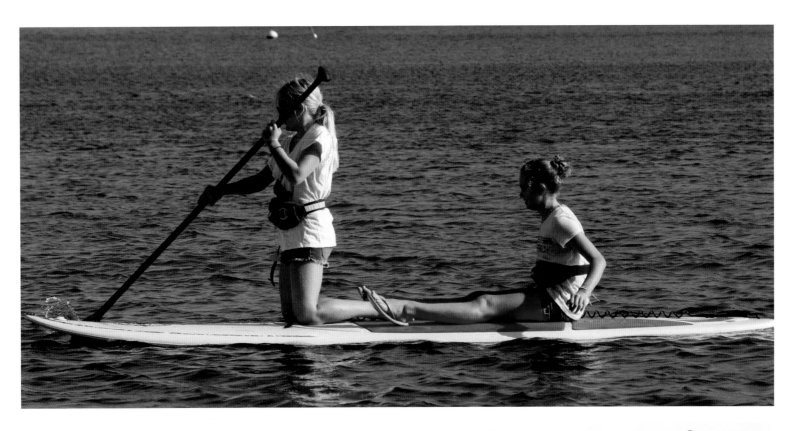

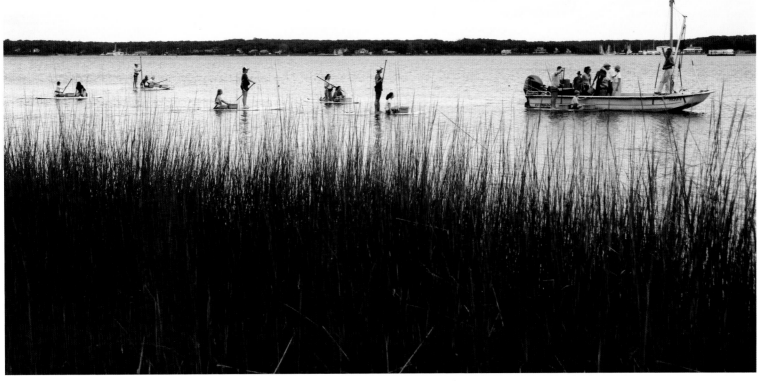

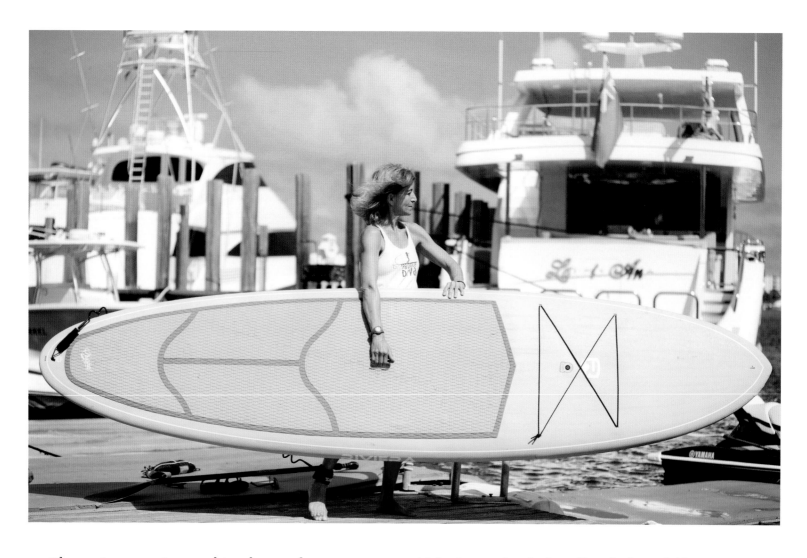

The environment is something that needs our attention now more than ever. It's becoming more and more important for all of us to take social responsibility for the world's oceans, as they are being more affected by human footprints and pollution than ever. The oceans and waterways need to be cared for and made stronger, much like our own cores as we paddle along them. I like to make the connection between the importance of feeling good about oneself and how that ties into being aware of our environment and the impact we have on it. There is so much in the press about global warming. Oceans and lakes with high nitrogen levels that allow for harmful bacteria to thrive cause the sea life to flounder and can prohibit humans from being on or in the water. It's nothing we cannot reverse, and we will. When the environment is healthy, *we* are healthy; it is just that simple.

When I opened the first Paddle Diva center, I had a student, Susan Rockefeller (who is now a dear friend), who had an enormous impact on my environmental perspective. When she first came to me for paddling lessons with her two teenage children, she explained that she wanted to stand on the water and feel what it would

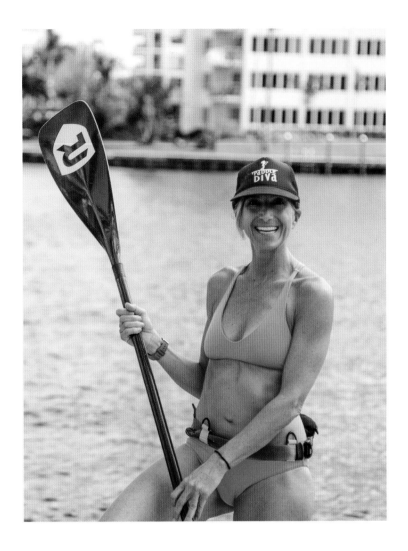

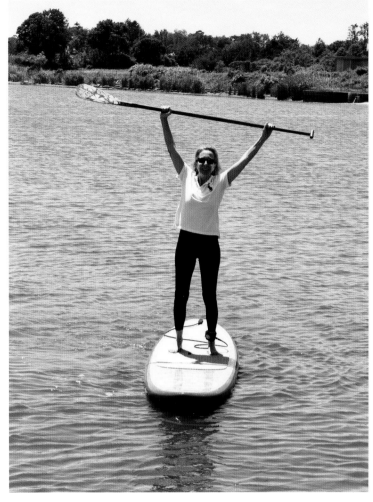

be like to use her own strength to power the craft. This was back in 2010, when SUP was in its infancy. Back then, we still got thousands of plastic bags when we shopped in the supermarket and used plastic straws in our drinks without any thought as to how these disposable, single-use plastics were polluting our precious oceans. If you wanted a reusable water bottle, you had to rinse and reuse the one you bought from the deli. At the end of our daily paddle sessions over the course of a week, Susan and I would sip from the plastic water bottles I kept in my cooler. She suggested that I consider offering water to my students using a less wasteful approach, like a water cooler and paper cups. A week later, I set up a water filtration system at my shop that took tap water and made it 100 percent potable. We were able to reduce our use of plastic water bottles. It was this tiny ripple of a suggestion that brought on a sea change inside Paddle Diva.

Later on, I worked with Susan on a documentary called *Missions of Mermaids*, a film she created using existing footage she had found on the internet and obtained the rights to use to demonstrate our need to let

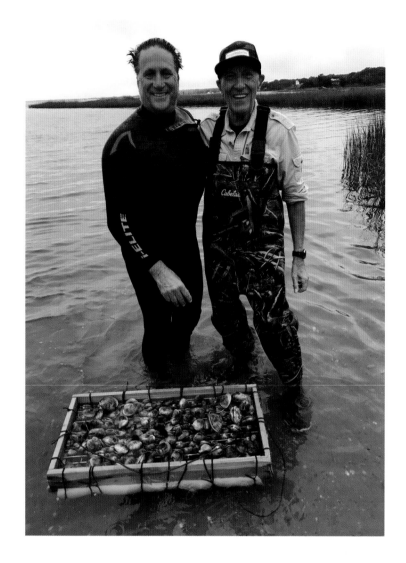

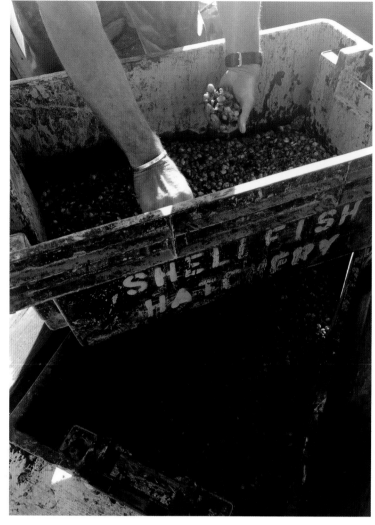

the oceans rest. I was so moved by the film and its message that I continued my conservation efforts and have become a proponent for clean waters in the bays of Long Island. Paddle Diva is a certified testing center for the Surfrider Foundation, a non-profit environmental organization that works to protect and preserve the world's oceans. In the off-season, we collect water samples and data from the bay to help understand how the effects of outdated septic systems and over-fertilization of lawns directly impact the nitrogen levels in our ground and seawater. We work with the Cornell Cooperative Extension. and the East Hampton Shellfish Hatchery to disseminate oyster spat (oyster larvae) and clam seeds. Most important, we work to clean up our beaches and answer any request for help with a beach or a bay cleanup.

I have had so many students who never thought about the impact we humans have had on the environment until they became Paddle Divas. Cate is one in particular. She had never paddled and bravely spent a

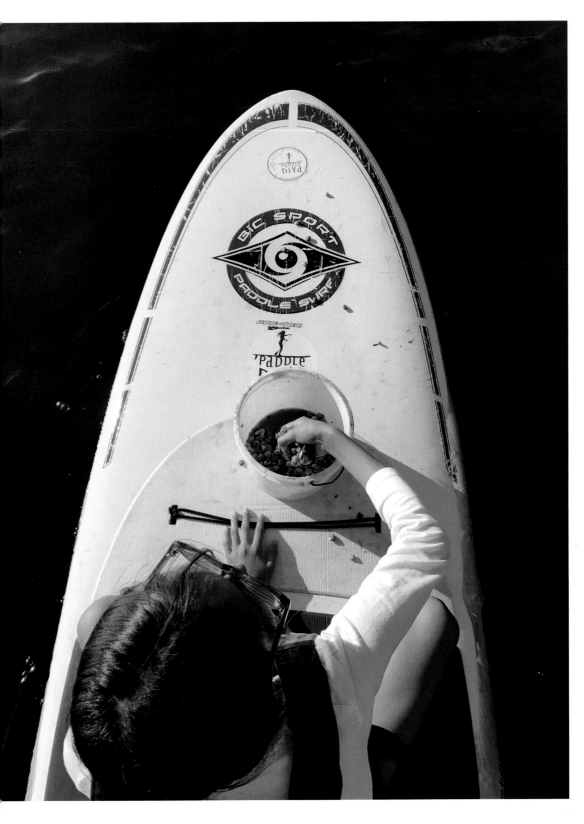

summer getting good at the sport. She spent plenty of time working with Shari, one of my original instructors who is known for her patience, and Mary, who is known for her persistence, to improve her stroke and stance and to build up her endurance in less than one year. She was so timid at first that the environment was not a focus for her, but as her strength grew from paddling, she started to look around at the declining waters around her. She got involved with the Cornell Cooperative Extension program and became part of its study to learn about the decline of the horseshoe crab population. She also serves with The Climate Reality Project, a group founded by former vice president Al Gore to promote an understanding of the realities of global warming. Cate is the perfect example of how becoming a paddler can build a strong core and then help Mother Earth protect her core. She became a paddler and an activist—a perfect combination.

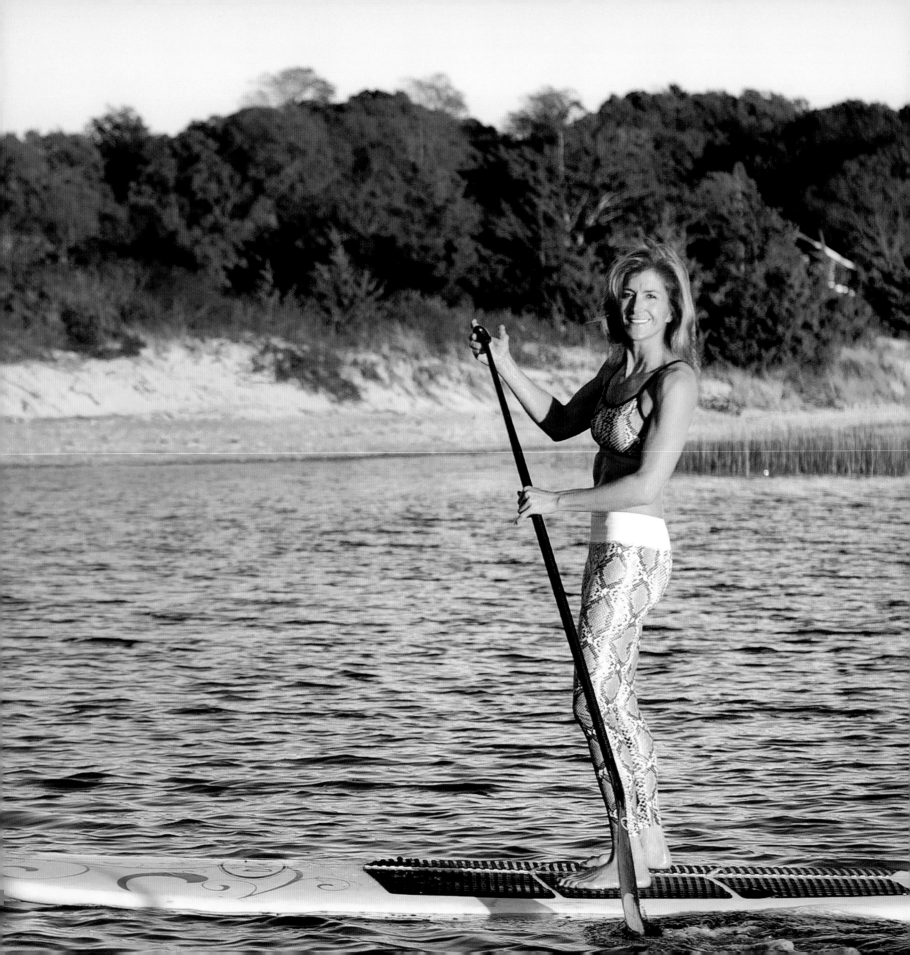

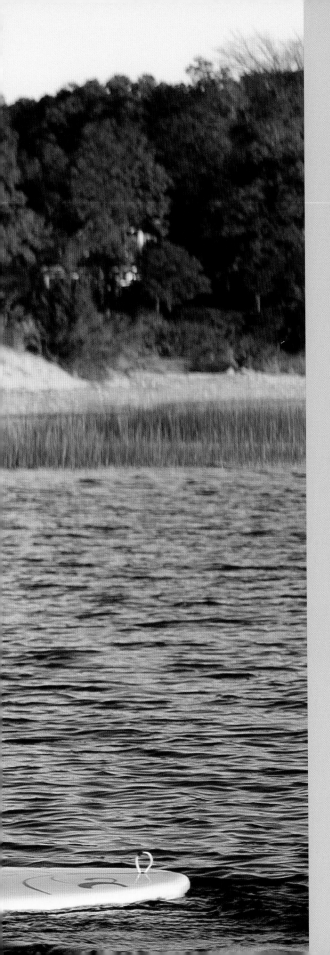

Enjoy the Ride

When you paddleboard, it feels like you are walking on water; you are using your arms and core to do all the work. The wind gently blows your hair back, and the cool water washes over your toes while your board skims the bay's edge. As you glide along, looking back at the shore, you begin to see the world through a whole new perspective. It's a full-body workout and a unique immersion for all of your senses. Whether you paddle out into the expansive bay or just explore cozy coves along the shoreline, each stroke of the paddle through the water puts you into a meditative state. You are on the ultimate ride, one you are enjoying and one that makes you feel content.

Early one morning in Montauk, just after sunrise, I met a group of women for an ocean lesson. We picked Gurney's, a historic oceanfront resort nestled in a pristine area called Hither Hills, as our launch spot so we could enjoy a green smoothie and frittata for breakfast before heading down to the water.

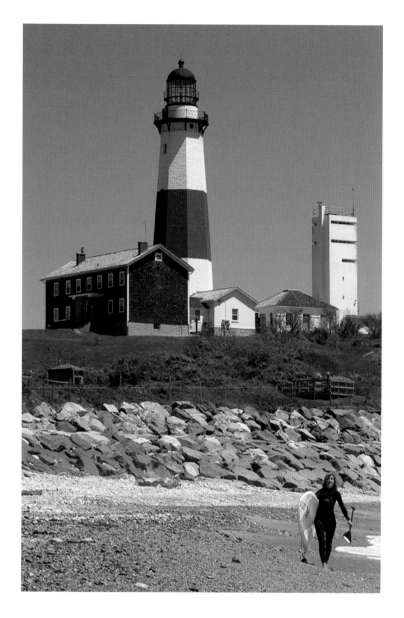

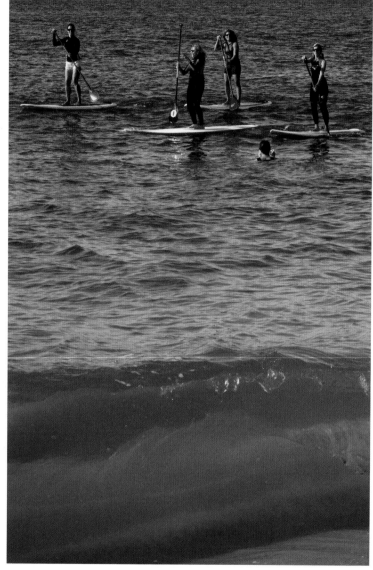

The beaches of the Hamptons are gorgeous, with dunes dotted by green sea grass that slope down to the white-sand beaches and dark blue waters of the Atlantic brushing up along the shore. There are hundreds of miles of bays and ocean beaches. One could explore for years and still find a new spot! On this warm, windless July morning the ocean was flat, with just a small wave at the shore that was easy to step over so we could plunge in for our morning pre-paddle swim. This was a great way to get my group of ladies acclimated to the cooler water temperature should we take a spill and fall off our boards.

The goal of this lesson was to get my students "out of their head" and to overcome their fear of the ocean. They were all nervous, and I just wanted to get them to enjoy the ride once we got out beyond the break. As we carried our paddles and boards down the cool morning sand, I

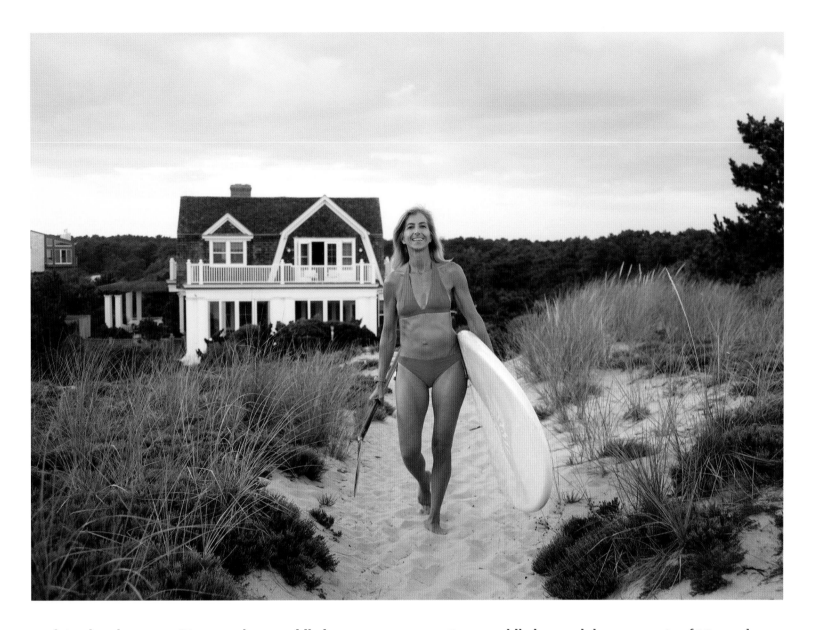

explained to the group, "Once we have paddled perpendicular to the waves and are outside the break, I want you all to take a moment to enjoy the ride. As we paddle along the coastline, keeping the beach close, you will feel the gentle rocking of the ocean and the current will make the trip out and back more challenging. This isn't about how far we go or where we end up; it's about the journey along the way."

As we paddled toward the eastern tip of Montauk, the sun rose higher in the sky and started to warm our bodies. As a group, we paddled quietly along at first, and I watched as each of the women started to relax, putting fear and expectations behind them. They were all living in the moment and enjoying the ride. I too just relaxed and took in all that I teach about. I stopped thinking about the day's appointments and where my kids had to

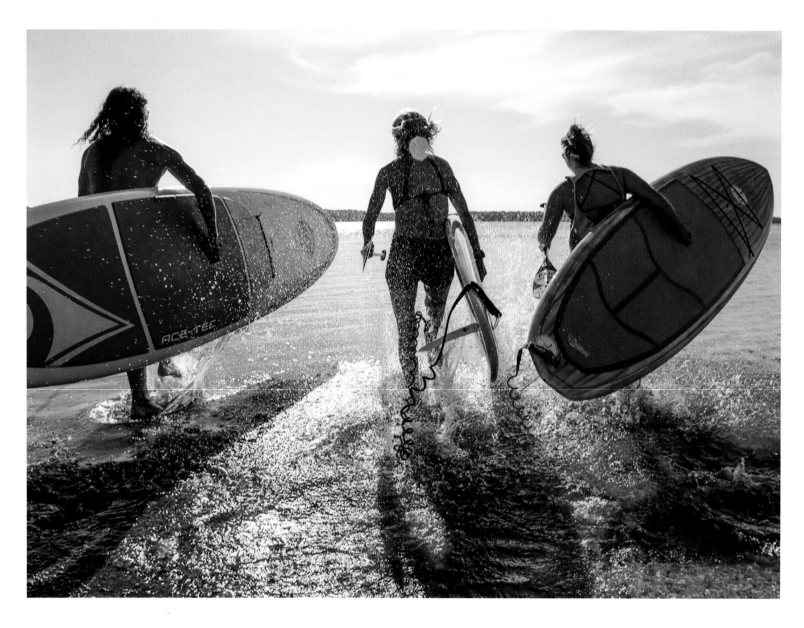

be driven to or from when I would be done. I looked out to sea; I looked along the white sandy shoreline at the large houses that emerged grandly from grassy dunes. This paddle, one of many more to come, was the point where we all had to let go and give ourselves permission to take the trip and have fun along the way!

One of my favorite fall paddles is when my veteran instructors and pure adventure athletes, Shari and Mary, and I take a group of hearty Divas and head west of the Hamptons. We hit the Peconic River to do what we call a "downriver paddle." We launch from Calverton and follow the river as it flows east right into the town of Riverhead. This is more of an adventure; it is truly the essence of "enjoying the ride." We take our Divas to a new place, out of their comfort zones; we have to portage our boards over roads and trails, and sometimes even have to briefly

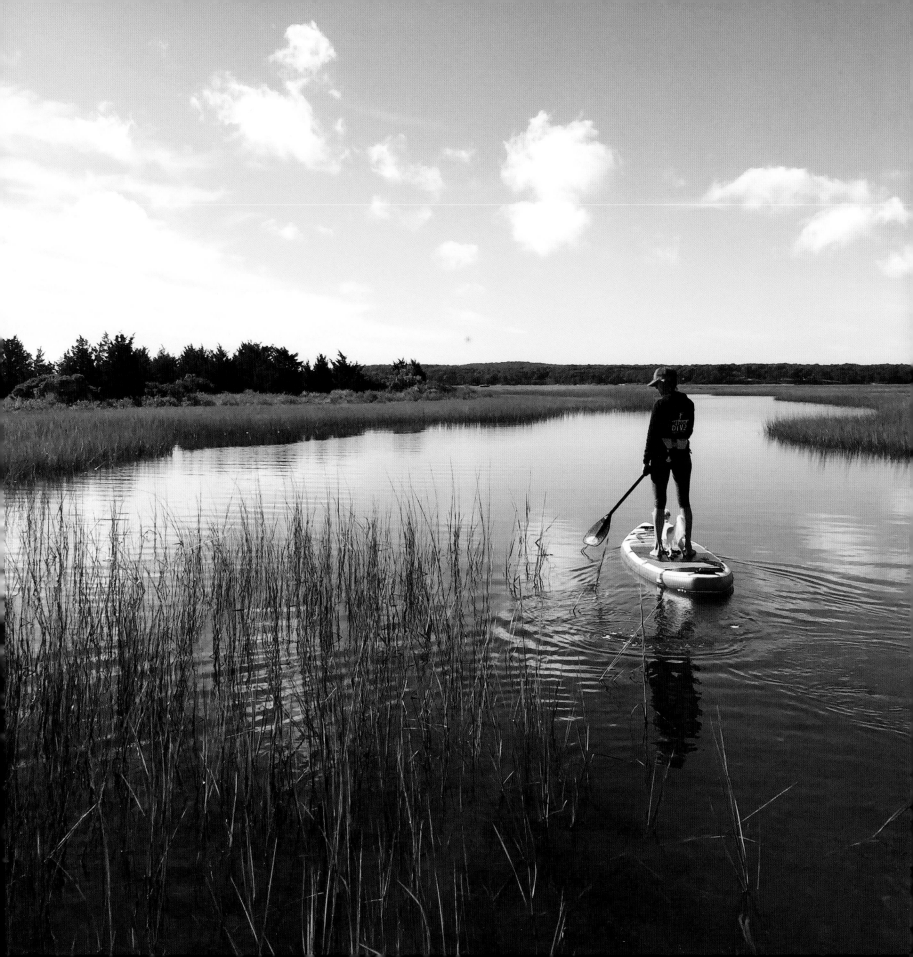

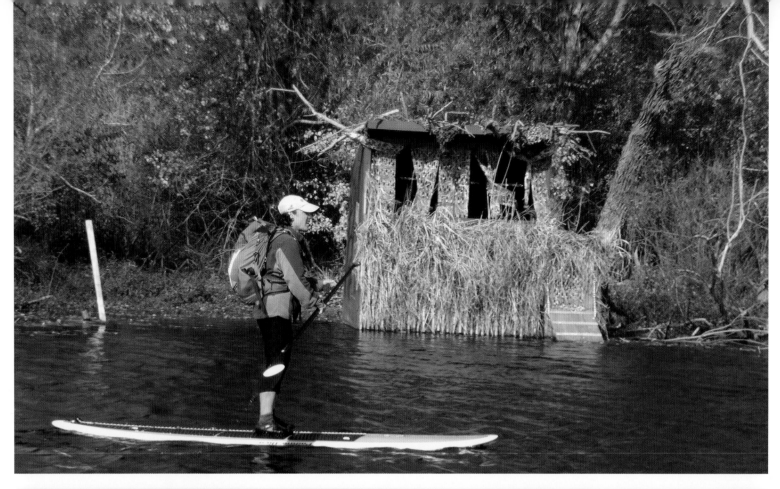

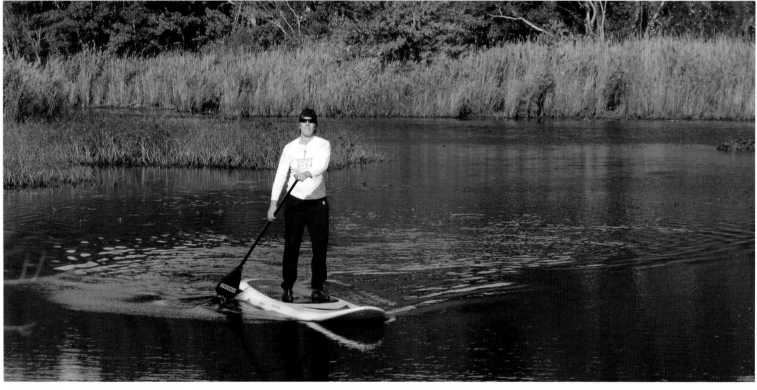

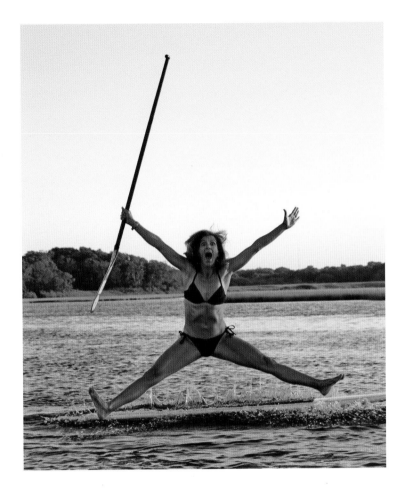

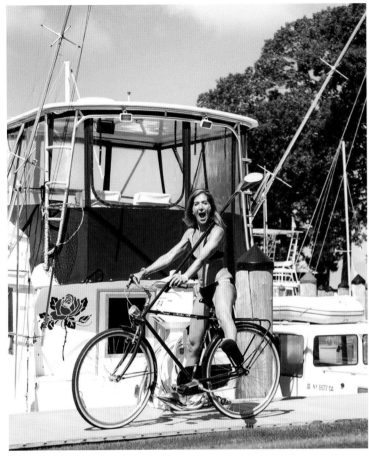

cart our boards through the woods. We have to go under the Long Island Expressway, through a wide tunnel that allows the river to freely flow and just pushes our boards along as we experience paddling in a way we have never before.

One November, I did this trip with a small group. We meandered down the river, and one of my regular students, Dianne, who gets anxious when there is no destination clearly in sight, kept asking Shari where we were going. I could hear the slight panic in her tone. Shari, who is probably one of the most empathetic instructors I have when it comes to helping women overcome fear, as she herself has used paddling to overcome her own fears

of wide-open spaces, is the perfect match for Dianne. "Dianne, just look ahead, to that corner. That's the destination for the moment." I looked back to observe. Dianne did exactly that but then said, "But after we turn, then where are we going next?" Shari artfully replied, "That's just it, Dianne. Keep watching for the corners, head towards them, and just enjoy this ride." In the cool autumn wind, my heart warmed when I saw Dianne's face after Shari's comment. Her expression lightened. She dipped her paddle in strongly and kept following along. She started chatting with Tim, another instructor along for the fun river ride, and I could see she was relaxed. She got it. Now she could just enjoy the ride. She glanced

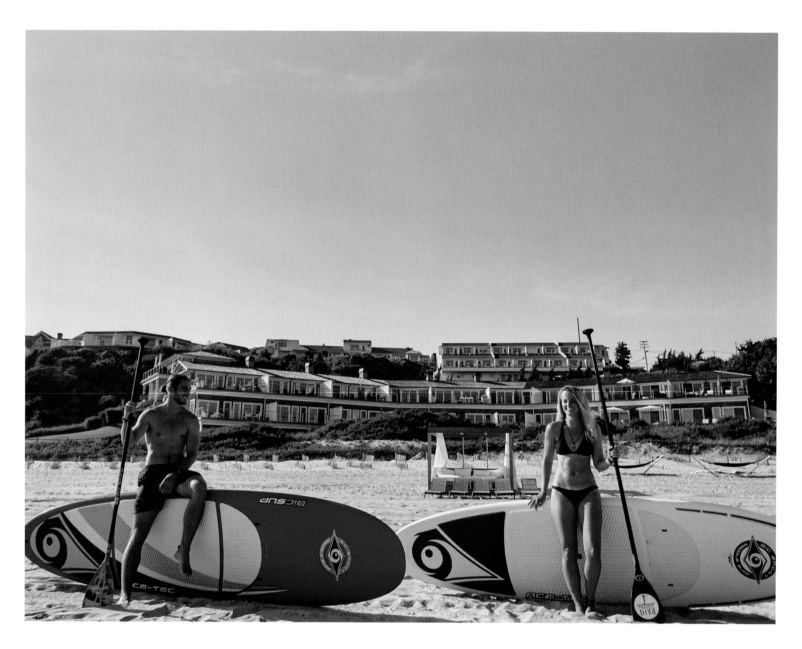

at each corner as we continued to wind our way down the river. As she and I loaded the boards in the truck at the end of the trip, I could see she was elated by her accomplishment. I asked her if she'd do this trip again. Dianne replied, "I am ready for whatever is next, Gina. I get it now. It's all about looking ahead, enjoying the moment, and not worrying about the end."

When I first started Paddle Diva, I had really big expectations for where and how this business was going to expand. I envisioned that Paddle Diva would be like the Starbucks of paddling—yes, I am ambitious. Imagine, wherever there is a great place to paddle, you'd find a Paddle Diva center and you'd have the same great experience wherever you went. I wanted to have my brand on

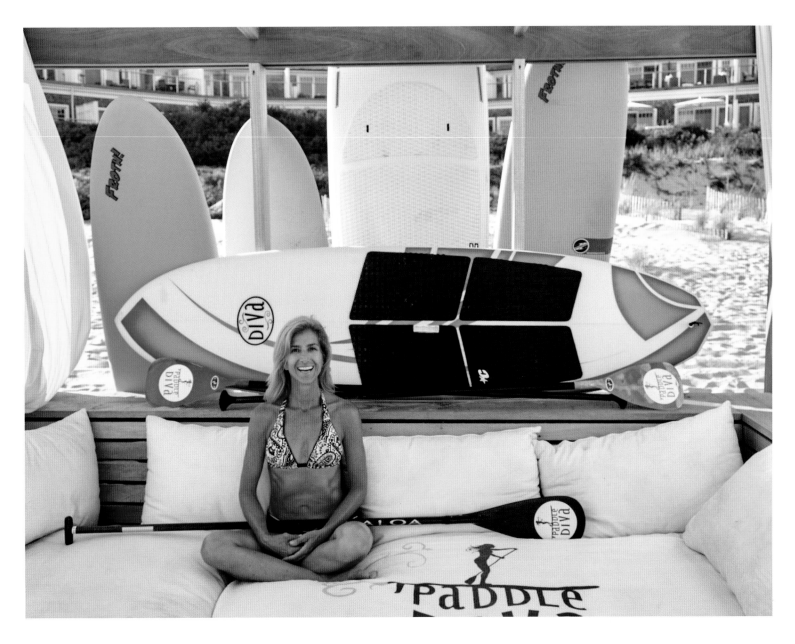

boards, wetsuits, and paddles and sell millions of Paddle Diva T-shirts and hats. I remember calling my sister and telling her I was going to start a business centered around paddling. In her very seer-like way, she advised me to just make sure I enjoyed the journey and to not worry about the end result. The journey is where you grow, learn, dream, and have fun. The end point is just that; it's the end. Now, ten years later, many of these things have happened and some have not, but the one thing that I can say with utmost certainty is I have consistently *enjoyed this ride.*

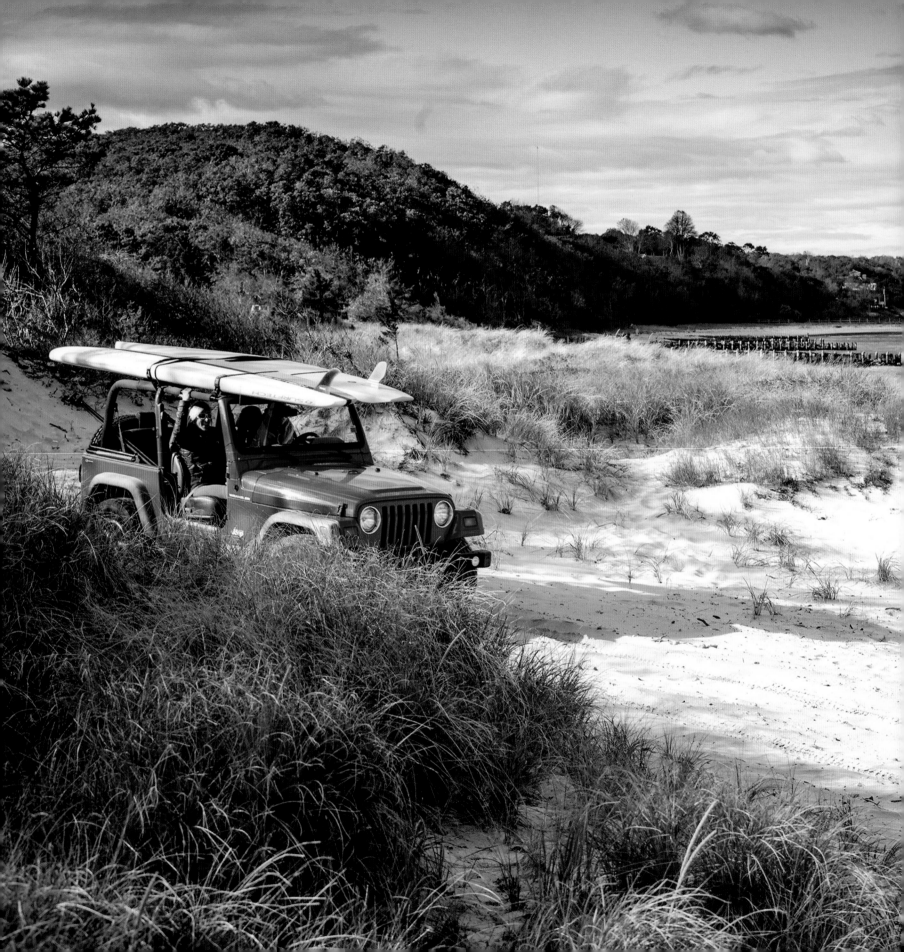

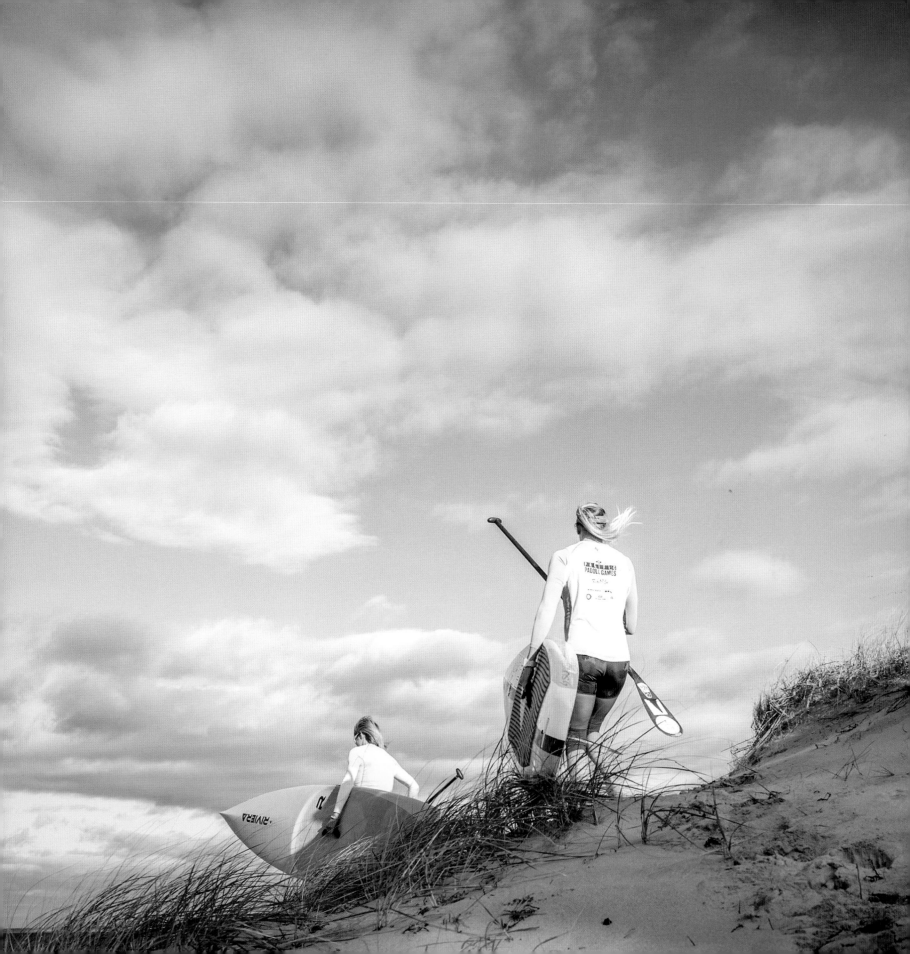

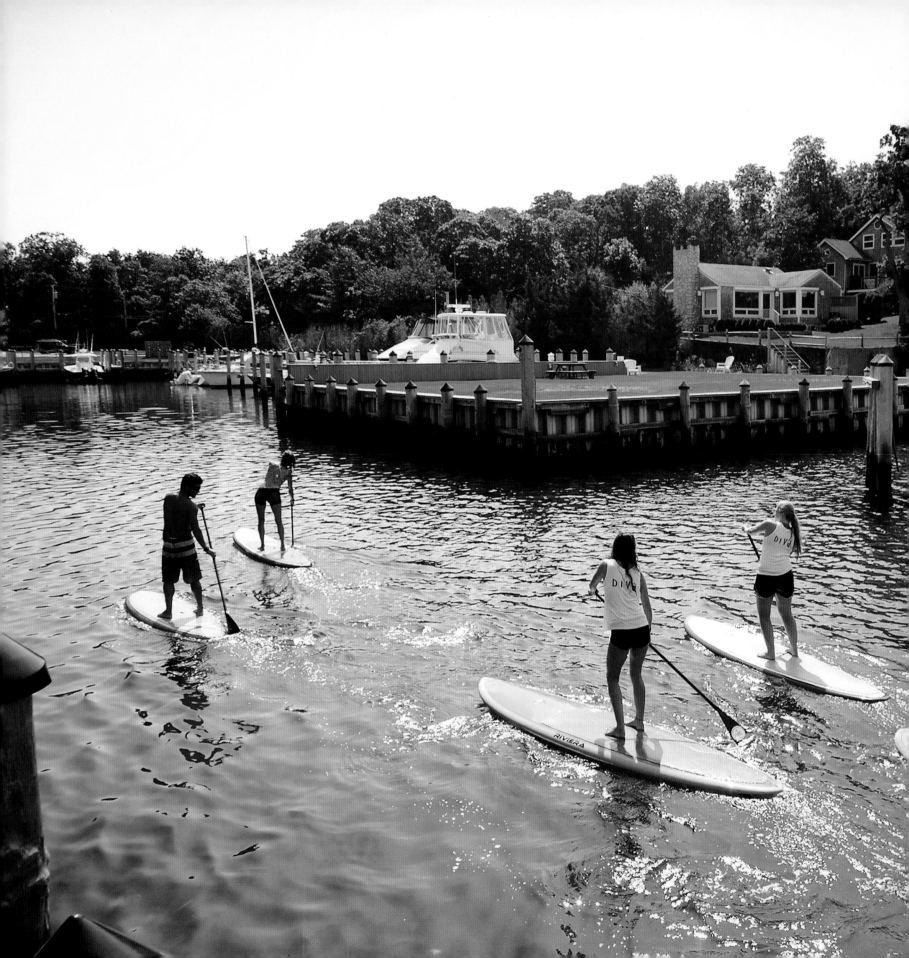

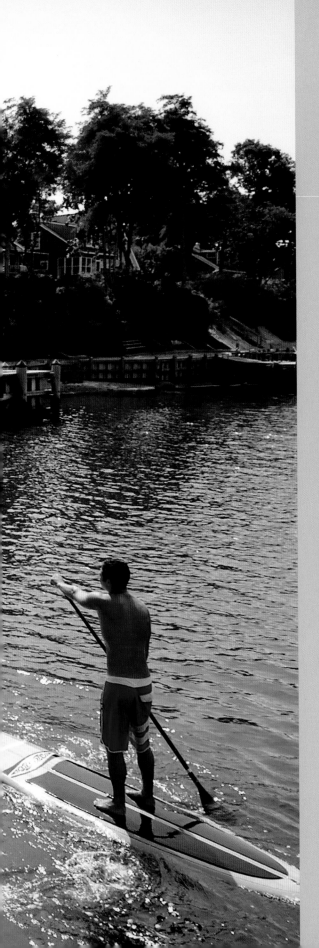

Be Comfortable with Yourself

"Falling in is just as important as paddling steadily on your board for miles," I explained to a group of first-time paddlers on a particularly balmy August morning at Paddle Diva East Hampton. "When you fall in, it allows you to cool off and learn how to get back up on your board. Most importantly, it will make you a more confident paddler. You will become more comfortable on the board because you see for yourself that you can handle any situation."

The Hamptons are famous for parties, fashion, real estate, and the natural beauty that surrounds the hamlets and towns that make up this coveted area. The Paddle Diva center nestled in Three Mile Harbor, just two miles north of East Hampton, is a refuge from the hustle and bustle of summer in the Hamptons. The minute you open your car door and walk across the gravel driveway

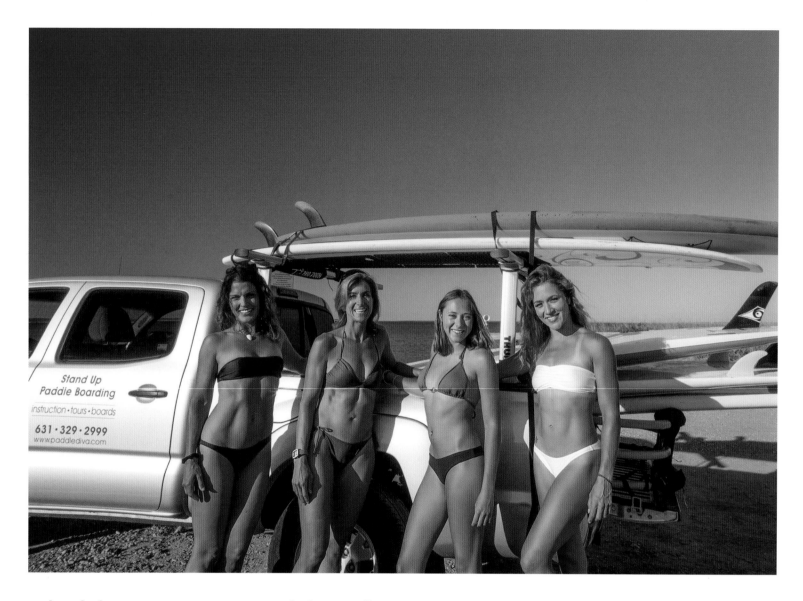

and up the brown steps to join me on my deck, you will know that you have arrived at a safe space. Paddle Diva is a place where you are welcomed, nurtured, and encouraged to feel comfortable with yourself. We welcome everyone and anyone who wants to become a member of our tribe. We are outside, where we all feel freer, enjoying the salty sea breezes and the gentle peeps of the ospreys. And this will be just the beginning of your life-changing experience with us!

One late summer morning, when it felt like it was too hot to even breathe, I had a group from a tech app start-up come out to Paddle Diva for a corporate outing. The goal from the head of human resources, who had booked this paddle with us, was to build camaraderie among workmates while learning to SUP. I was delighted because building people's comfort with themselves on a paddleboard is a great way to show them that they can do the same thing on land. Paddling forces the issue of

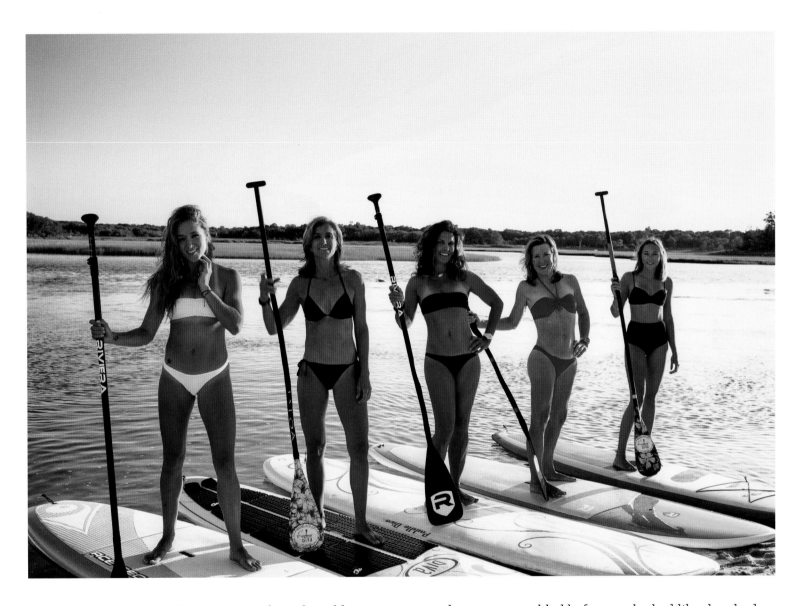

getting comfortable by allowing you to be vulnerable in a bathing suit, flopping into the water if you fall off the board, and wiggling yourself back up and then standing and being part of the group again. When you disembark from the board at the end of a paddle with your group, you all have that experience to share because you all succeeded in this one thing: stand-up paddling. You now feel that kinship, and your comfort level on land with yourself automatically increases.

The gang assembled before me looked like they had all spent too much time looking at a screen under the glare of the fluorescent lights of their office. Not my typical group, but I was excited to work with them. They came in all shapes and sizes, but all the students clearly possessed the feeling of being okay with who they were as they emerged one by one from the bathrooms, out of their urban street clothes and in bathing suits, showing off their white skin that had obviously not seen the sun

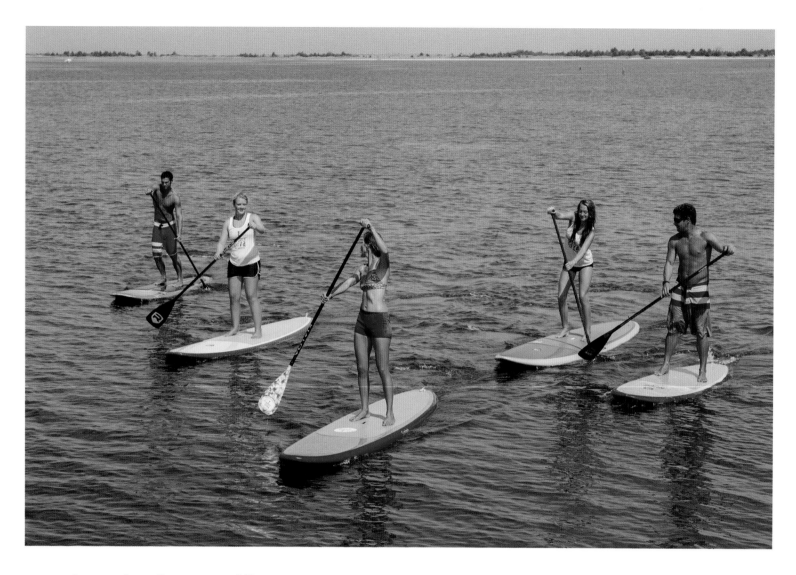

in months! But they all were at Paddle Diva to try something new.

As I do with beginners anytime we start out, we all stood in a line and faced our boards out to sea. This makes it easier for beginners because they are looking out at the horizon and can't compare themselves to the others around them. The group slowly went from kneeling to standing at different times, and eventually they were all paddling. As we glided along the bay for our hour-long journey, we all laughed and enjoyed just being out on the water.

Being a Diva means you are okay with how much you weigh, you have good self-esteem, and you are happy with where you are in life. When you are a Diva on the water, you have the sense that you are fine just as you are and you are truly comfortable with yourself. Paddling takes away the need for comparisons, and in this intimate marine environment, as you stand proudly on your board, you don't ever feel the need to do things simply to impress others.

When we paddle, we provide all our clients with the option of wearing a PFD (personal floatation device). We

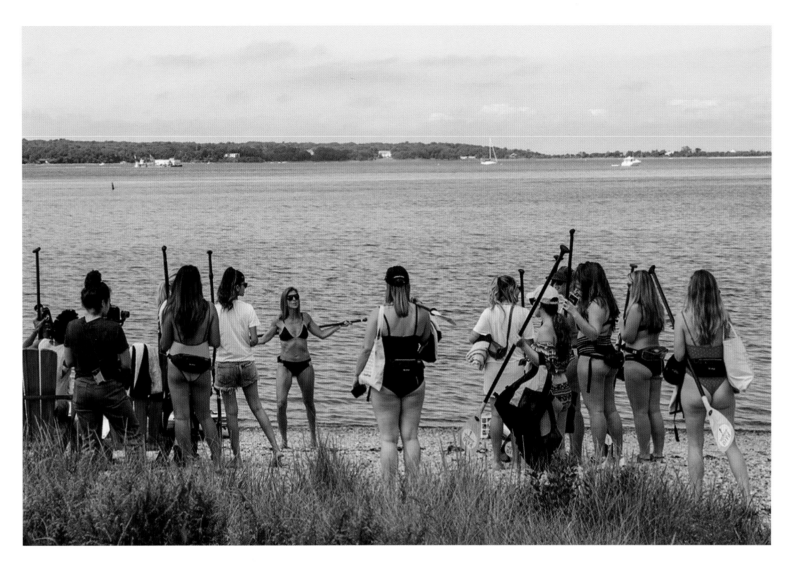

have plenty of life jackets and life belts; if you pull a cord on your jacket, it automatically fills with air to float you. Given these options, and the fact that all students are required to wear a ten-foot-long leash that attaches their ankle to the board, they often pick the life belt because it just feels less cumbersome, although if you fall in, they will not float you! What I admire most, however, is when I have students who want to feel the comfort of the extra safety of the jacket and wear it without caring what anyone else thinks. I have one advanced student, Karen, who paddles every day and smartly chooses to wear a life jacket. Not only is she showing me her commitment to the sport, but she is also demonstrating her own ability to not care what she looks like and paddle with the safety of a life jacket. By always choosing to don a life jacket, she inspires potential students who think they cannot paddle because they are not strong swimmers. That is someone who is truly comfortable in her own skin and can stand apart from the crowd and wear a life jacket when everyone else in our group wears a lift belt. While this

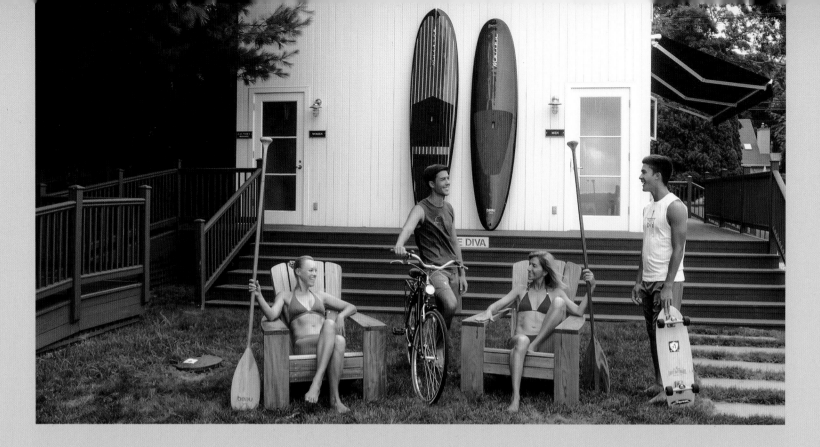

How a Paddle Dude Can Become a Paddle Diva

By Tim Wood

It's 8 a.m. on a brisk sunny morning in late spring when I show up at the Paddle Diva center for the first time. Gina stands at the top of the stairs contemplating a broken paddleboard with concentrated amusement. She looks up, swoops down, and greets me by name. Gina is ebullient and wants to get out on the water right away. It feels like we have known each other forever. I came to Paddle Diva two years ago to get certified as a SUP instructor; I stayed at Paddle Diva because I loved its mission and Gina's vision. Since that day, I've seen many people's lives transformed by learning to SUP at Paddle Diva. I've even seen dudes transformed by the experience, which gets me to the elephant in the room or, in this case, the elephant on the paddleboard.

Many clients look at me funny because I'm a guy wearing a Paddle Diva t-shirt. Personally, I've never really had a problem with the fact that Divas are usually women, and dudes tend to be men. But let me be clear: Women can be dudes, and men can be Divas. For a dude, paddleboarding is just a leisure activity. But for a Diva, paddleboarding is a high-intensity workout, an emotional journey, and a spiritual exercise. Getting trained by Gina quickly revealed to me that paddleboarding takes brains as well as brawn, humor as well as concentration, gratitude as well as grit. So how can a paddle dude become a Paddle Diva? Here are five key things I learned as a Paddle Diva instructor that might help you get there.

Paddle on and have fun!

1. **Divas don't give up.** Paddleboarding looks easy, but it takes endurance, practice, patience, balance, commitment, and a willingness to get wet! Dudes can have a hard time with the fact that paddling is harder than it looks and can give up rather than lightening up and having a good time.

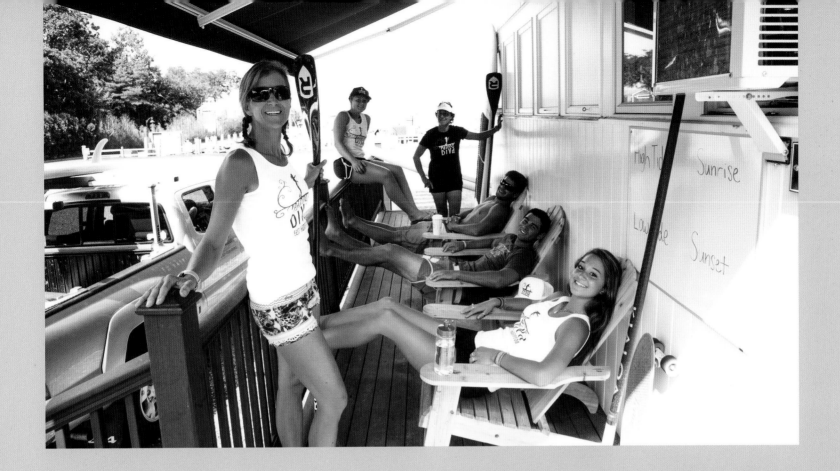

2. **Divas know that anyone can paddle, and paddling is for everyone.** Divas create an inclusive space free of judgment and full of encouragement. In order to become a Diva, a dude needs to leave the competitive ego behind and get stoked about the way paddleboarding brings everyone together.

3. **Divas know that you don't have to stand to paddle.** Dudes are too concerned about paddling the "right" way—that is, standing up—rather than paddling well—which means feeling good while paddling. If you're having fun sitting or kneeling, then you're paddling the right way; if you are not having fun, even if you are standing up, then you need to change the way you are paddling.

4. **Divas fall!** Everyone takes a plunge once in a while. Dudes worry about falling, and it messes up their balance, not to mention their good time. The best thing a dude can do to improve balance is actually fall in because it extinguishes worry and fear. As any Diva will tell you, falling isn't failing. Getting wet is one of the greatest pleasures of paddling!

5. **Divas know how to be in the moment.** The point of paddleboarding is not to get somewhere but to be where you are when you're there. Look around, paddle away, and get lost in this one particular beautiful day on earth!

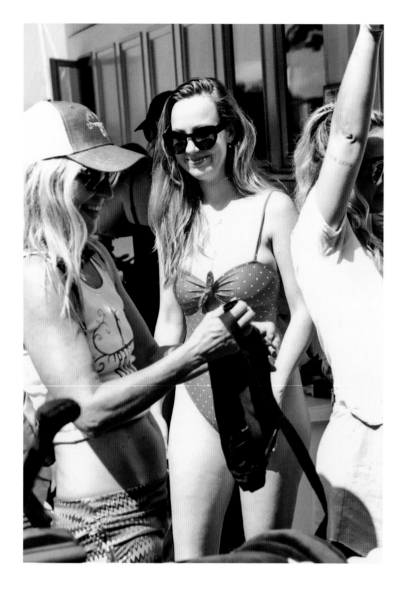

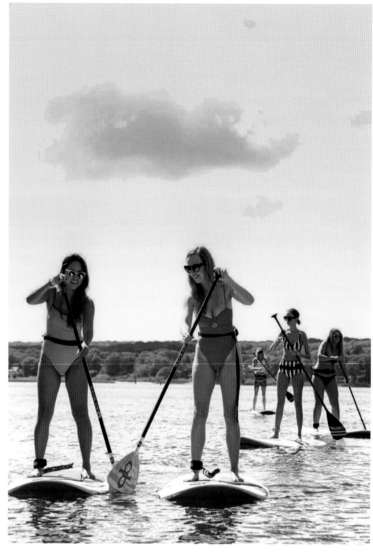

may seem like a small detail, her braveness to show that this is what she needs and she will wear it proudly is the epitome of feeling comfortable in your own skin!

Karen has used paddling to help her overcome many personal issues through her advancement in the sport. She had thought about paddling for a long time but thought she could never do it well. At one point, she was a great windsurfer, but had suffered from health issues and thought she'd never find her way back onto the water

to ride the waves again. Karen and I spent hours building her strength and courage as we paddled through every possible condition. Over the years, Karen has paddled her way into feeling comfortable with herself and her image on the water. She's one of the most enthusiastic paddlers you will ever meet. She has made me a better leader and teacher, as many students can do. Karen has tested my ability to differentiate and modify a lesson; she has pushed me to hone my skills as a teacher and pushed me

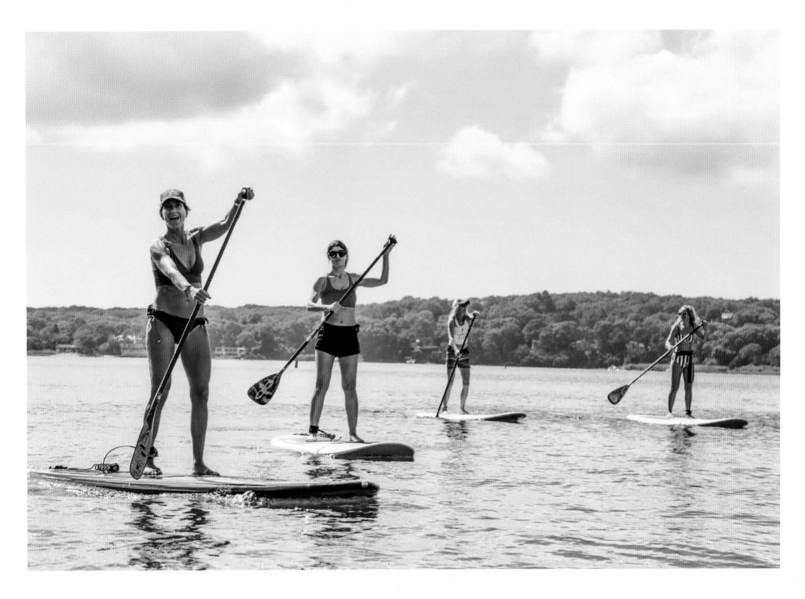

to be a leader. These are absolutely the best students to work with, and her pushing me to improve is exactly why I loved my hours on the water with Karen.

Since Karen and I met over five years ago and started working together, if asked, she will tell you that paddling saved her life. She has gone from the bays of the Hamptons to the harbors of New York, where she paddles by the *Intrepid* with my dear friend Eric from Manhattan Kayak.

She has raced in the Paddle for Pink on the Paddle Diva Team, finishing in the top ten. She gained a great new confidence as she went from a beginner to an advanced paddler, and this confidence shows itself on land as she moves through her days, waiting for the next chance to paddle.

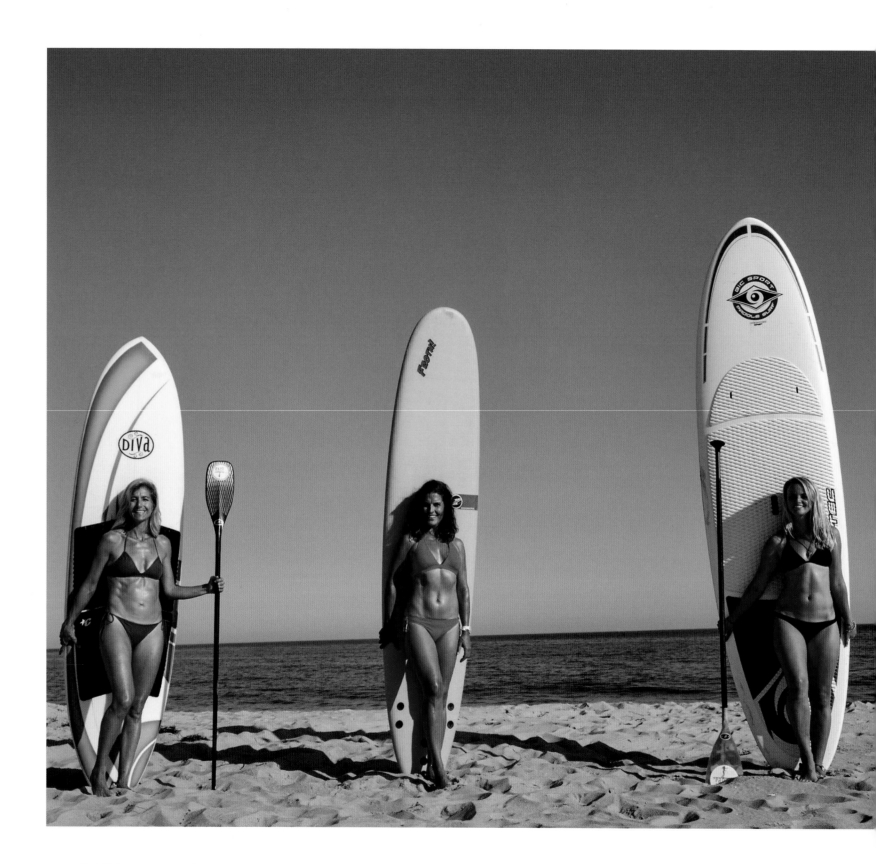

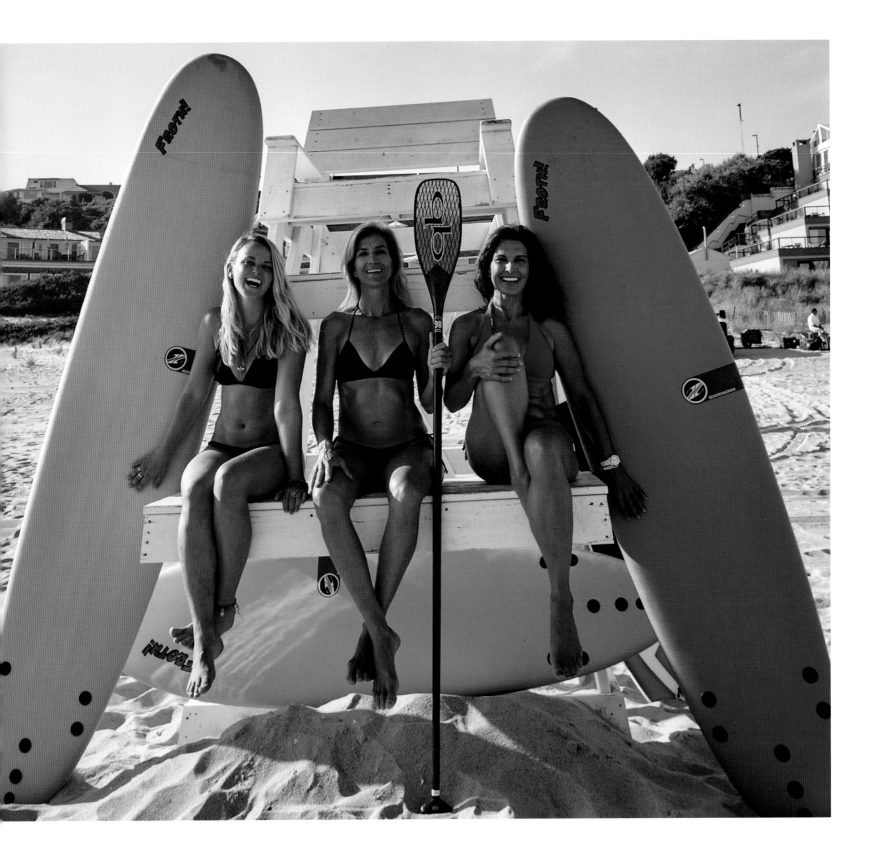

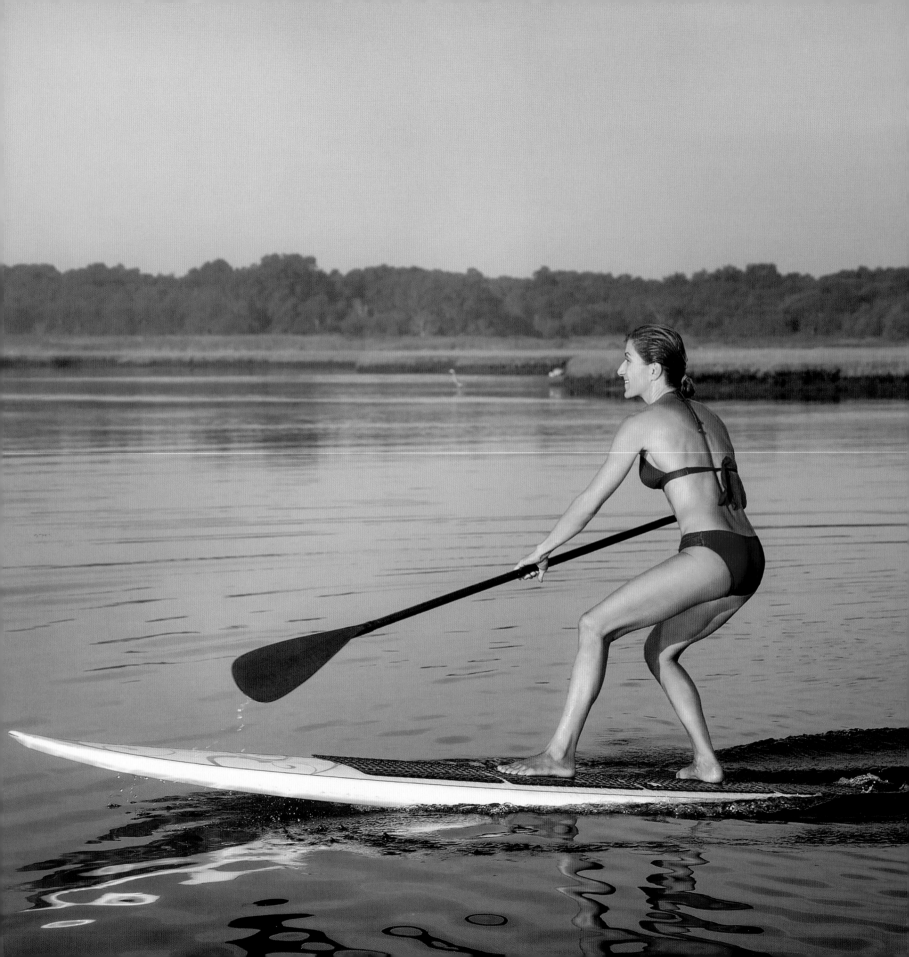

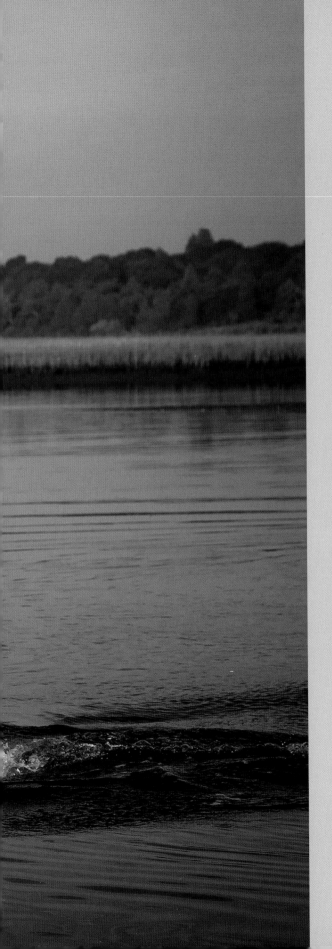

Move (Gently) Outside Your Comfort Zone

"We begin and end every paddle from a kneeling position," I explained to a class of beginners gathered in our secluded cove at the Paddle Diva center at the Shagwong Marina. I demonstrated the move and then explained, "As soon as you stand, you are going to feel a bit awkward and your legs may shake. It feels wrong to be standing in the middle of water, but you have to ignore what your brain is telling you and gently push outside of your comfort zone."

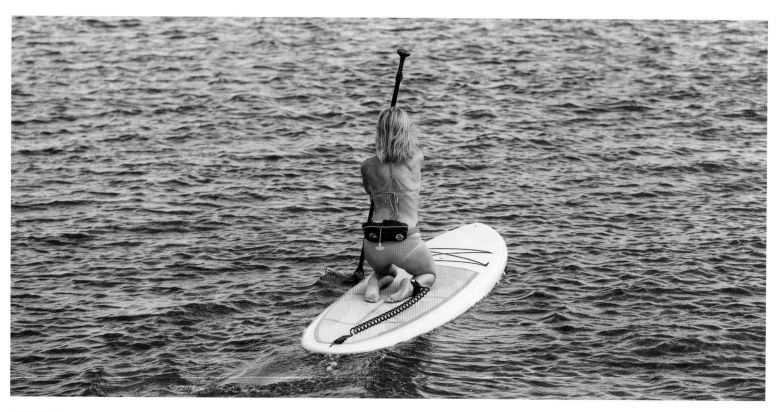

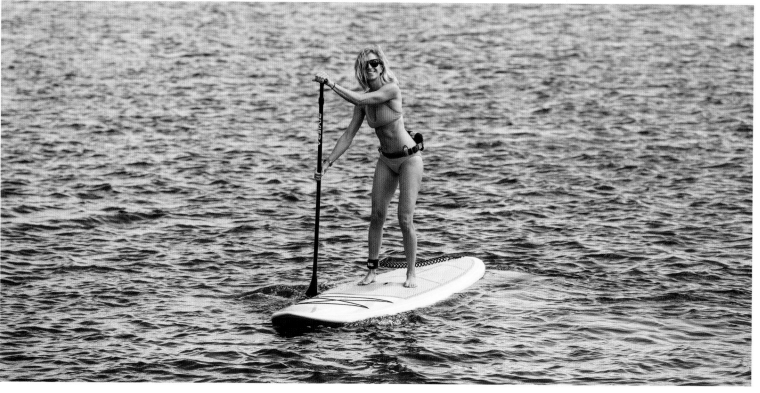

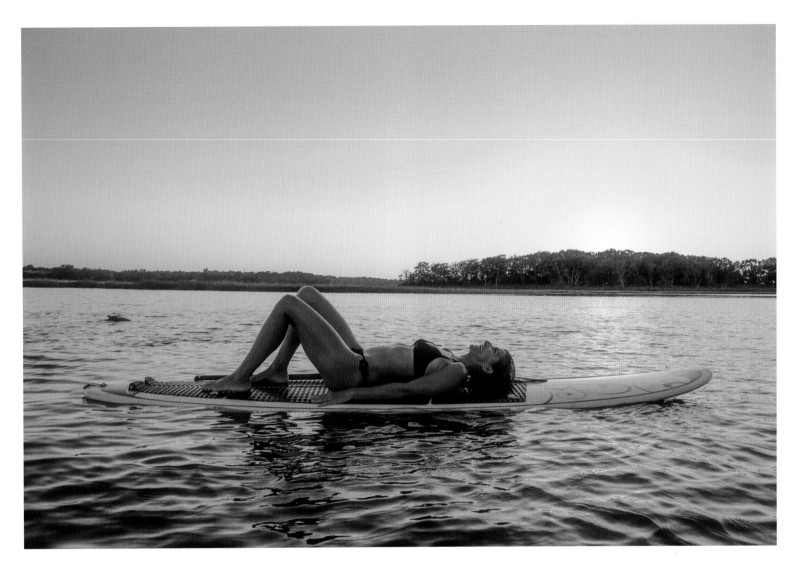

Often, when students first learn how to SUP, it's the most real way they can push themselves out of their comfort zone. Some students are afraid of plunging into the dark water. Some students get anxious at the thought of falling behind in a group paddle. Some fear that their muscles will fatigue or they will hurt themselves. However, by the end of that first lesson, most of them will find that their whole mentality has changed because they have learned how to move along the surface of the water and overcome the fears they had at the beginning of their first lesson. From the moment they paddle off from the shore, they are committed. They have no choice but to continue, and along the way they often find that their mental barriers become broken down by the serenity of their surroundings. They have learned that you can push outside your comfort zone on the water, and they begin to imagine what they could do on land, if they just tried.

Three years ago I was asked to host the paddling session at Gabby Reece and Laird Hamilton's XPT Experience. This three-day life-changing event takes place at

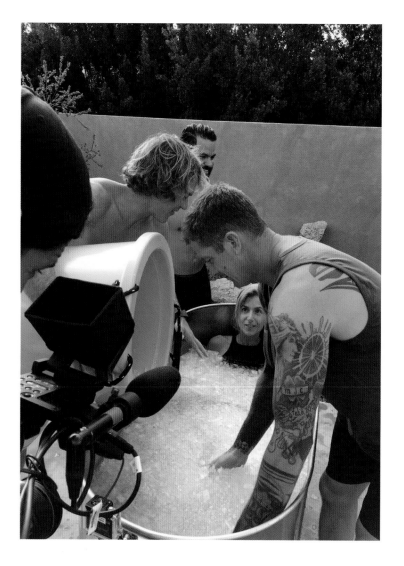

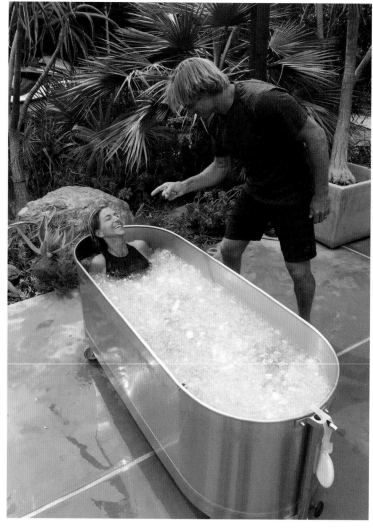

locations all over the globe. Led by Gabby, Laird and their team, participants are taken through the breathwork, ice and heat recovery, pool workouts, and mobility training that allow us mere mortals to live our active lives without injury. The moment you meet the team, you immediately fall in love with this group of intelligent, experienced, and humble leaders in fitness, surfing, and recreational sports.

This three-day experience showed me how I could hone my mind skills and pushed me out of my comfort zone in the pool workouts, in which we wore snorkel masks and did underwater drills with weights in the pool. I was guided in immersing myself in an ice bath, followed by a hot sauna and finishing off in the ice bath again. I had to repeat over and over to myself, *I can do this*—or, as Laird always says, "This is my home; I live here," as he plunges into a three-minute soak in near freezing waters. It's an experience to be done only in the presence of leaders like Laird and Gabby. As I kicked along the deep end of the pool, I'd surface to the sound of Gabby's voice saying, "Great work, Gina. Now, do it again!" I'd inhale

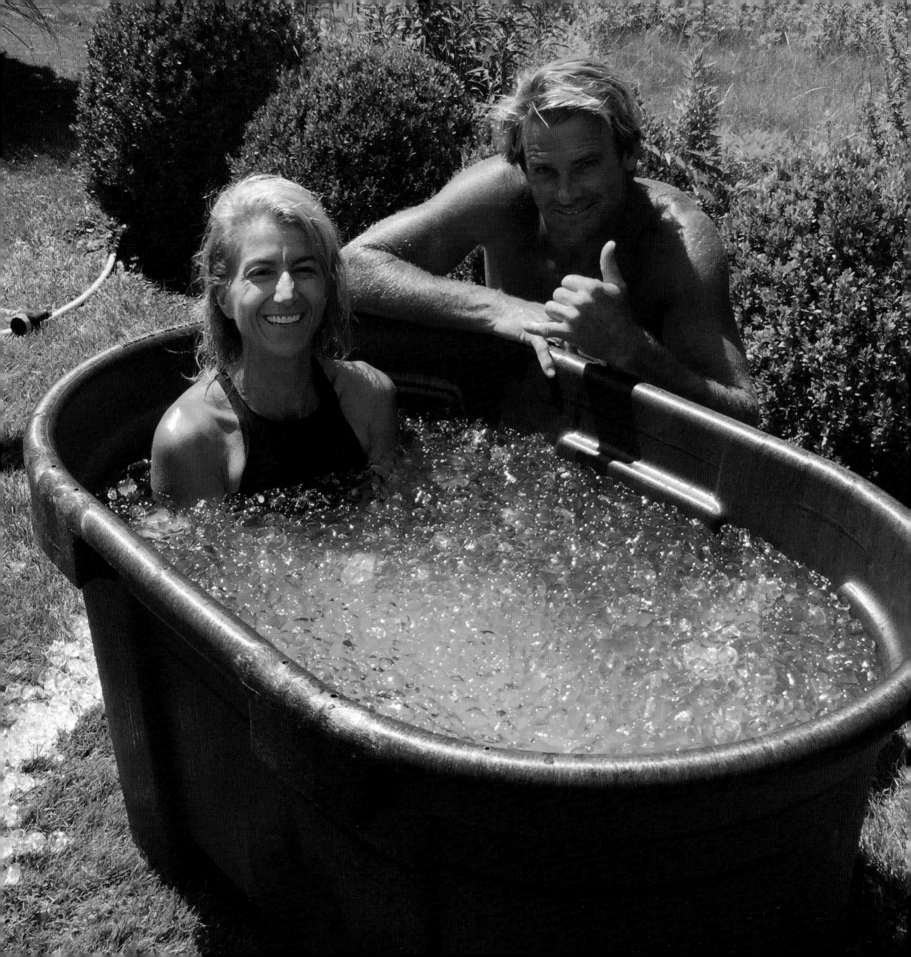

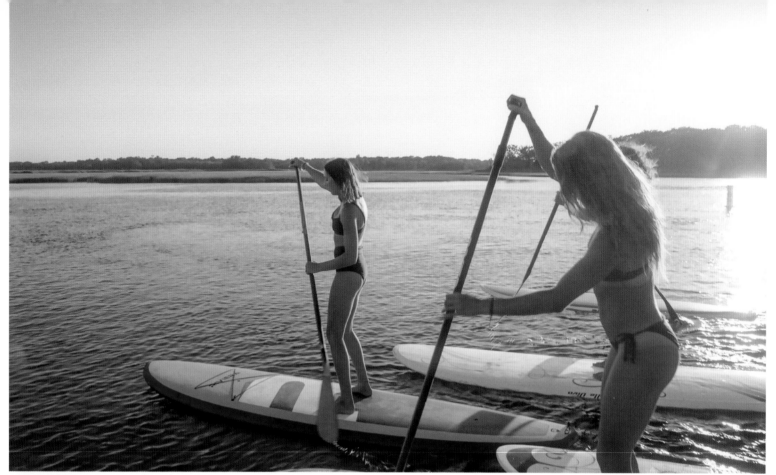

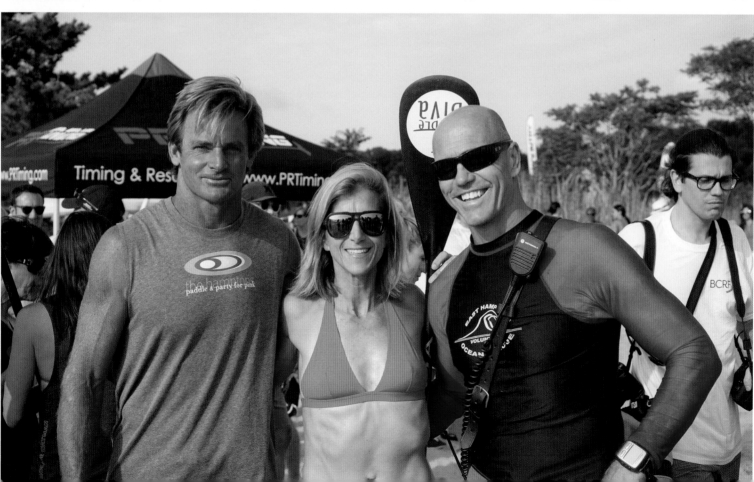

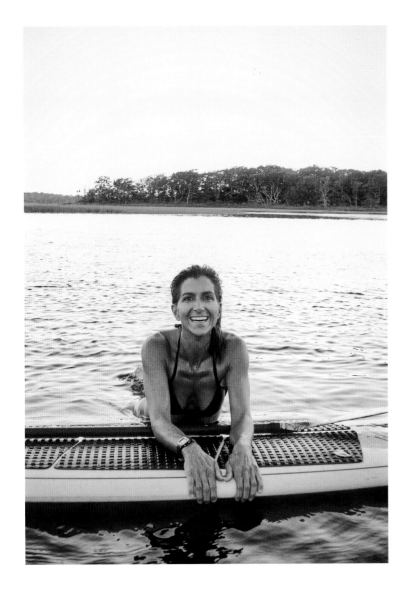

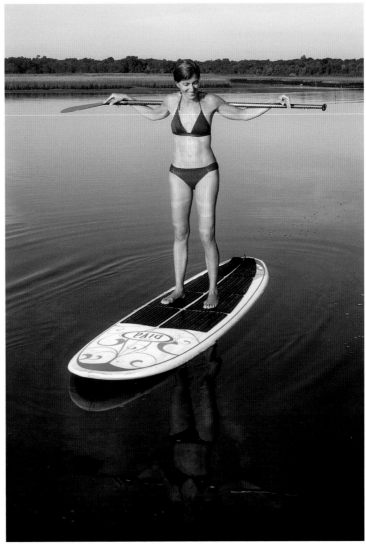

deeply and head back across the pool, never breaking the surface because my mind was allowing me to be pushed outside of my comfort zone. I had never felt so good!

I recall one student, Andrea, now a dear friend and an avid paddler, who watched me instruct Paddle Diva classes for three years from her houseboat before she agreed to a SUP lesson with me. She had all sorts of objections. Her shoulders needed strengthening. She was scared. She did not think she could do it. She would fall

off. And, one of the most common ones I hear, she had bad balance. (Side note: If you can walk, you can paddle.)

When I finally took her and her husband, Allen, out for a paddle she was elated by how fast she learned, how easy this sport is and, most important, that she pushed through her internal objections. Now she is a proud stand-up paddler! Andrea is one of the tribe. She now sends me pictures of her paddling all over the country. Having her own passion and developing her identity as

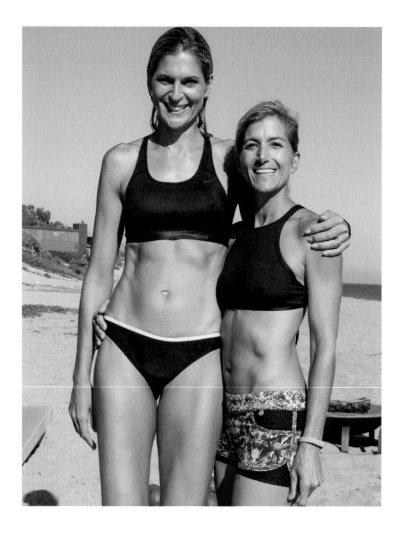

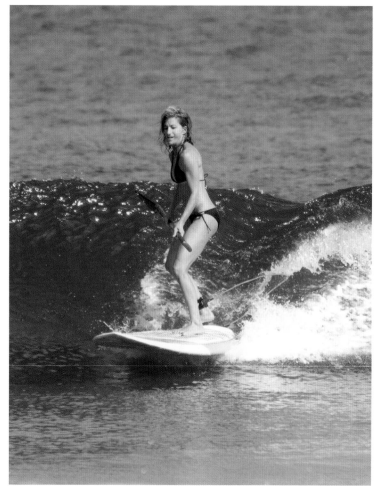

an experienced paddler has even added to her already amazing relationship with her husband. She often nudges him to join her on the water when they are traveling or at the Paddle Diva center where they keep their boat. Their shared passion for stand-up paddling adds to their quiver of activities they love to do together.

On land, we face obstacles and potential pitfalls every single day. It's so easy to let fear freeze our progress. I'm not talking about taking huge risks or doing anything dangerous. This is about engaging in small acts that gently nudge you out of your comfort zone, and that will ultimately crack open a world of new experiences for you. Getting married, graduating college, starting a new job— every new stage of life gently moves you outside of what you once thought was comfortable and into a world of new possibilities.

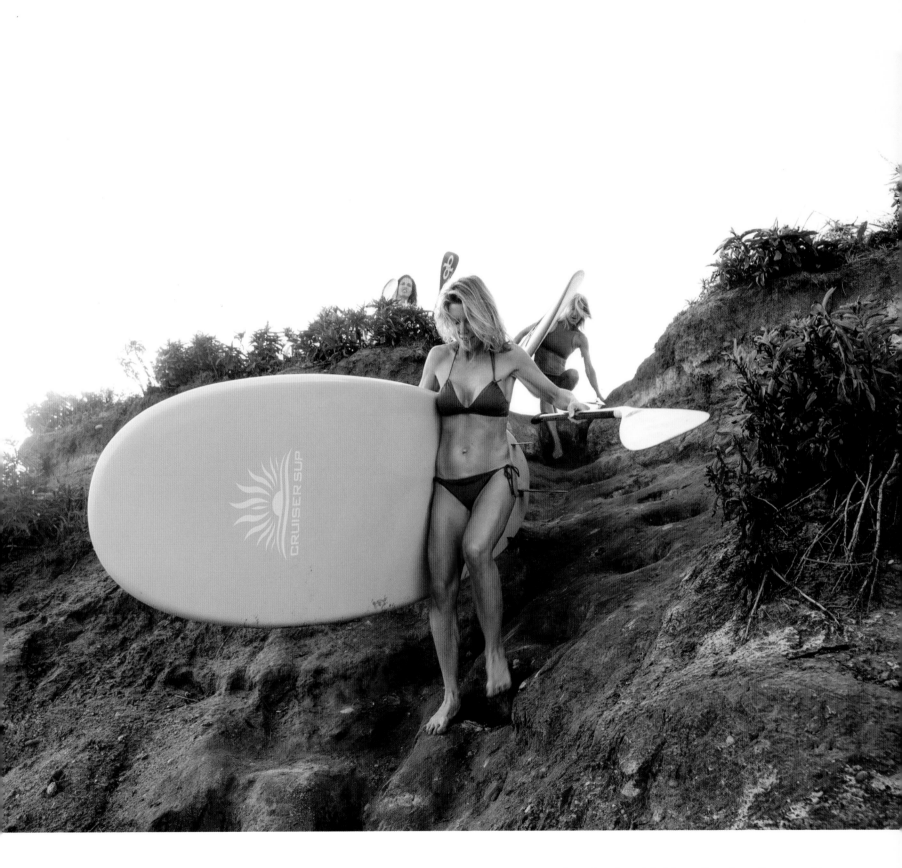

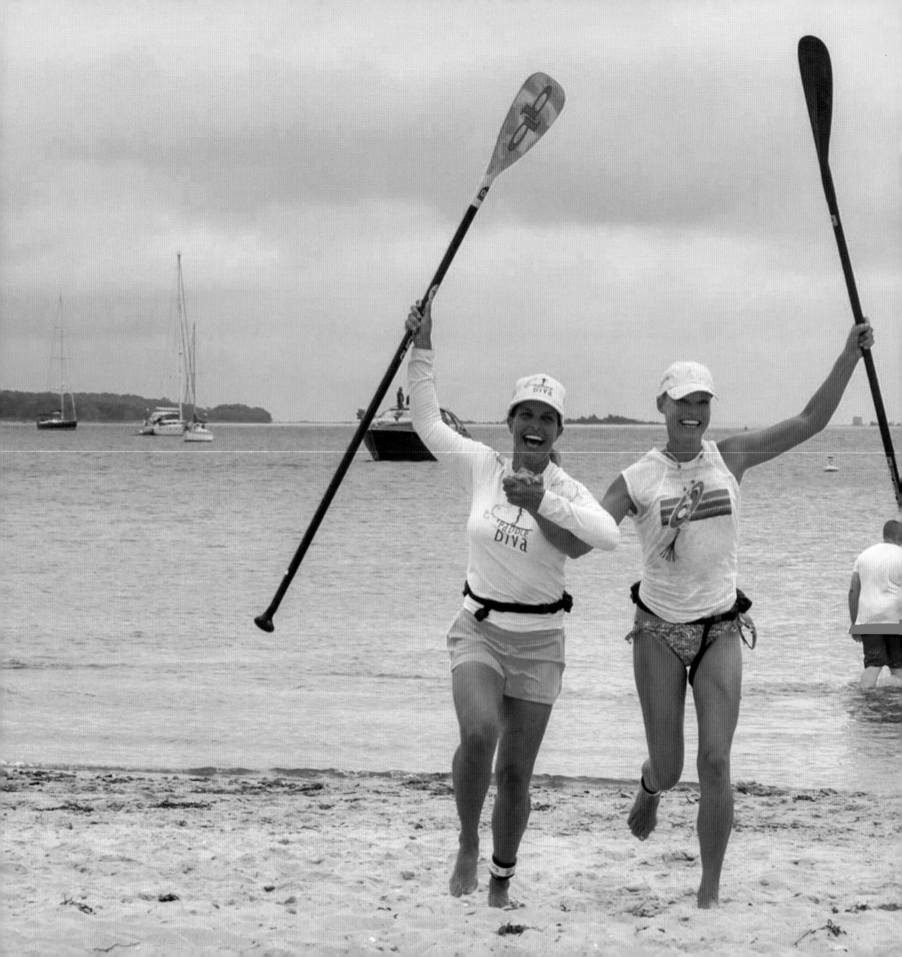

Positivity Is Contagious

"We've got this!" I encouraged Team Paddle Diva one ominously overcast morning at Haven's Beach, Sag Harbor in the Hamptons, as we prepared to compete in the Breast Cancer Research Foundation's annual Paddle for Pink race. "If I'm going, you're all going. I know we can do this, and I will be with you on the water for the entire course. I know you all have what it takes."

Racing is a fun aspect of SUP. I especially love doing it when there is a cause attached. On this day, we were working with community stalwarts Maria and Larry Baum to raise money for BCRF. Races are a great way to see how positivity can run rampant in a crowd. It's contagious! The finish line of any race is probably one of the best places to spectate if you want to feel uplifted. As a racer you have one goal: getting to the finish to the cheers of the crowd.

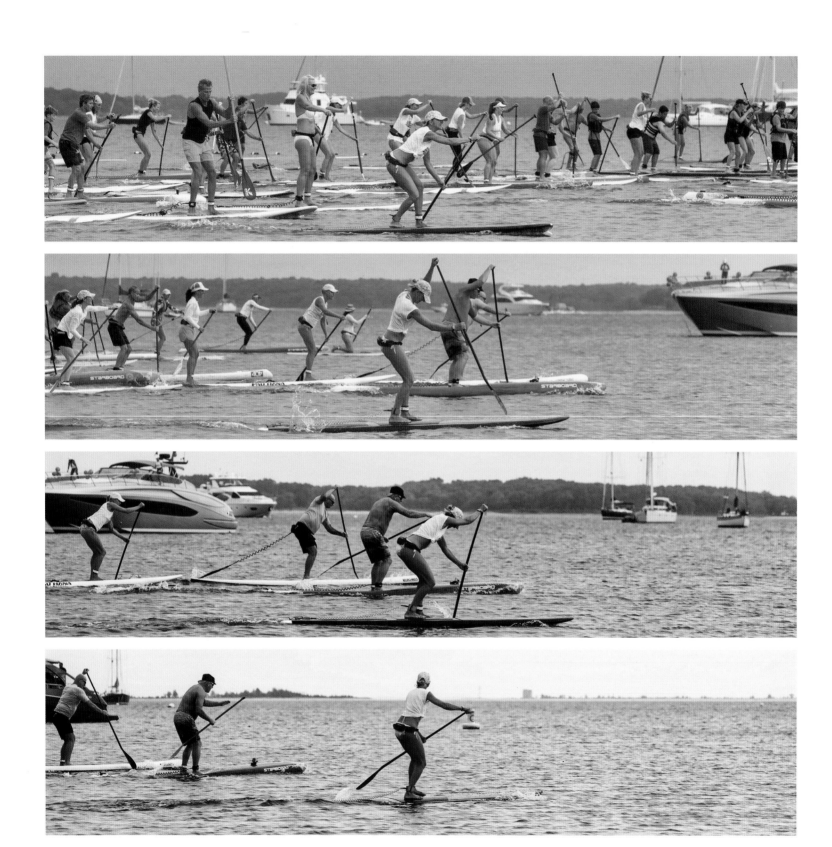

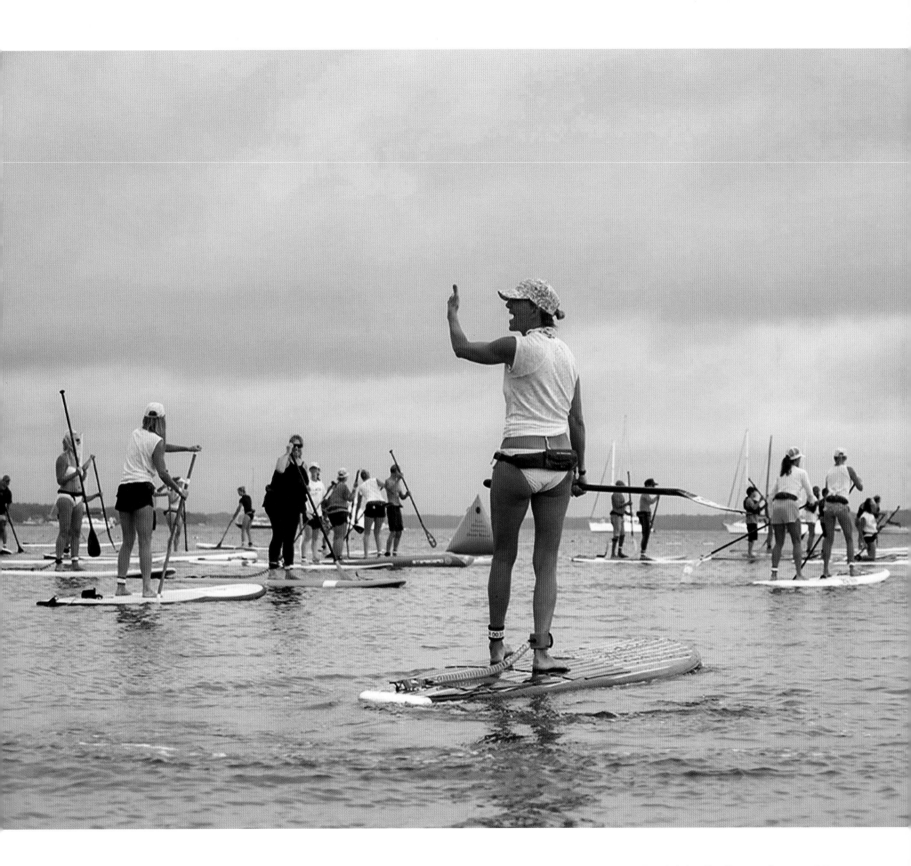

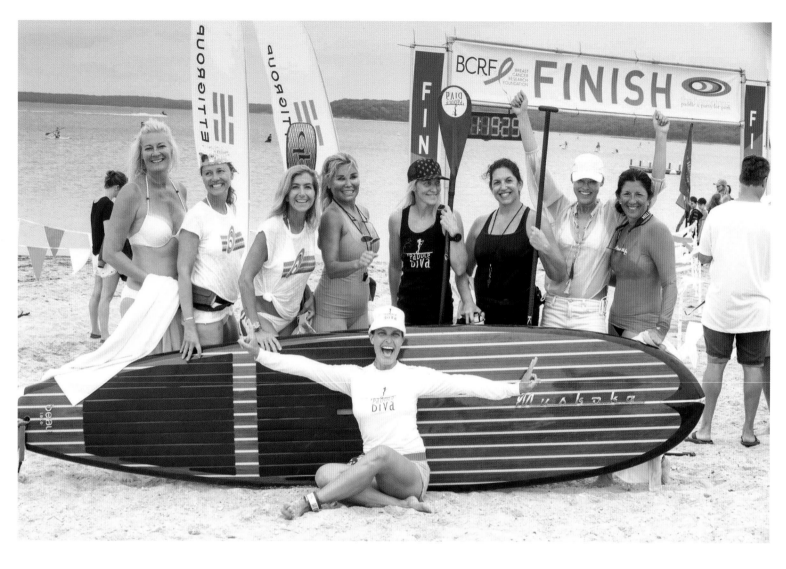

On this early Saturday morning, it took only a few words of positivity to lift the cloud of anxiety that loomed heavily over the racers as they anticipated what lay ahead. Lars, from Main Beach, the local surf shop, was on the loudspeaker hyping the crowd and encouraging the 150 male and female competitors to get ready, get set, *go!* As soon as the horn rang and the crowd cheered and roared with excitement, I could see the nervous energy of my team shift to positivity as we all pulled our boards through the water over the starting line. Like raindrops on still water, the crowd was filled with joy and excitement, and we paddlers were filled with energy and paddled on!

As we all paddled through the three-mile racecourse, I broke out in front of the pack to lead the ladies through the course so they could clearly see what buoys to turn around and how to best position themselves so they would have an easier time on this cloudy, windy day. As a beacon for the crowd behind me, I was showing the group that they could make it to the finish line: *If* I *can, then* you *can.*

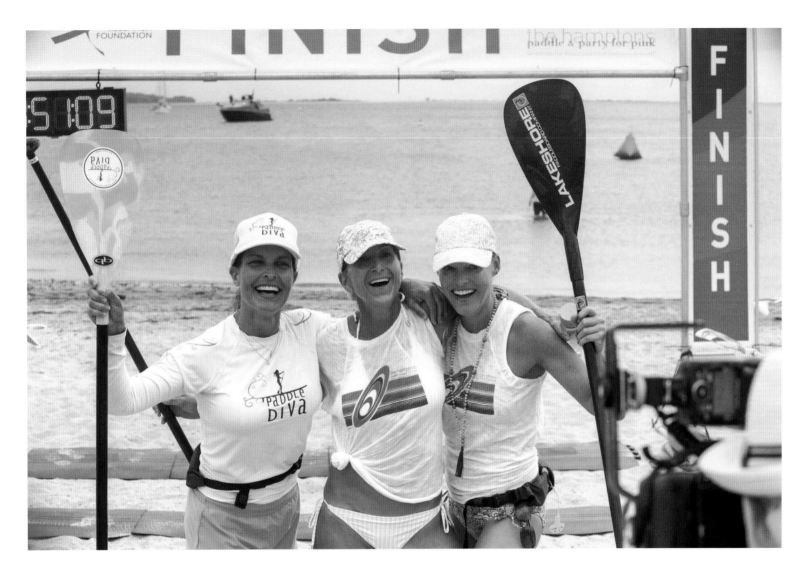

Two of my teammates, Jennifer and Helen, had decided to do this particular race on a tandem board. This type of board is built to hold two people, so it's longer, wider, and more buoyant than a typical board. It's also a really fun way to paddle with a friend and learn how to communicate so you paddle fast and in sync. Jennifer, a breast cancer survivor who used positivity to fight her cancer into remission, has done this race on a tandem every year since her diagnosis to show that overcoming breast cancer is a team effort. It's a journey that one does not do alone! Jennifer, one of my dearest friends and my first "guinea pig" as I tested out how to teach SUP (in 2008), has taken so much of what she learns and does on a board and brings it right back on land.

When Jennifer felt a small lump on the right side of her breast two summers prior to this race, she thought nothing of it, but a cancerous tumor was quickly revealed, thanks to Stony Brook Southampton Hospital's Ellen Hermanson Breast Center. Jennifer's attitude from the first diagnosis to her remission was one of a positive

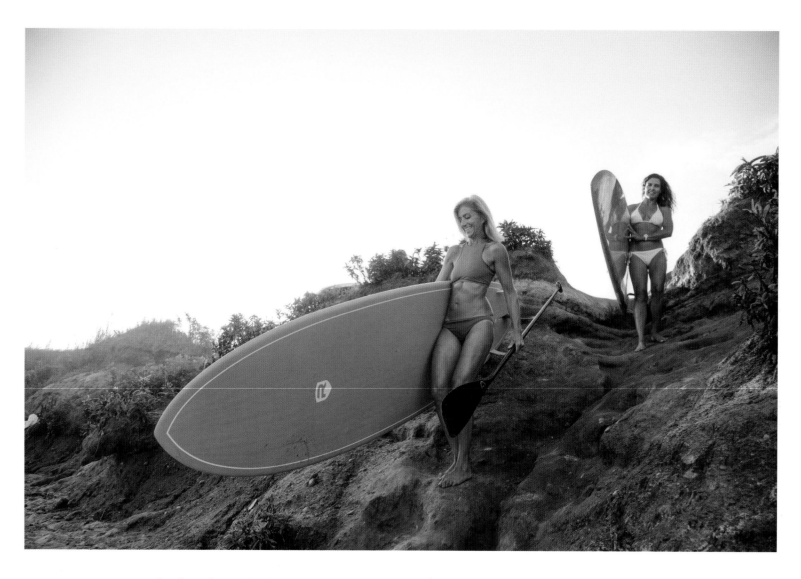

survivor. As soon as she found out she had cancer, she was ready to wade through the morass of medical choices to educate herself about all of her options and emerge a joyful victor in the removal and rebuilding of her breast. She never used negative words like *struggle* or *fight*. She never defined herself as a victim or even as a patient. Instead, she educated the people around her with her version of the disease, which she took incredibly seriously, but she also kept things joyful and filled with laughter at the appropriate moments.

I believe that part of Jennifer's two-year journey as she rid herself of any potential cancerous cells and recurrences with such a successful outcome was due in part to her positive attitude the moment she heard the words "you have cancer." Jennifer has also learned and grown so much out on the water as a paddler. She has remarked many times that she went back to how she first felt on a paddleboard and the power and the positivity she felt out on the waters with me as we took our water journeys when I was first starting Paddle Diva. She felt invincible

Origin of the Divas

By **Jennifer Ford** (mother, cancer survivor, and lifelong Paddle Diva)

The moment I met Gina it was as if the universe was reminding us that we were long-lost sisters. Our bond was instant and natural. Fifteen years later—years of massive transformations for both of us—our friendship is enduring and very precious. Gina has been by my side as I have gone through ending a marriage, raising a son with autism and a precocious daughter, and suffering as a single mom through breast cancer.

Gina and I were both busy moms who loved fitness and being in nature. When we were both lucky enough to get a sitter to watch our kids, we'd head straight outside, regardless of the weather, for a long run. One day, running through the woods, we came upon a brackish lake, and Gina said, "This would be a great place to paddle!" I assumed she meant kayak paddling, but she said, "Stand-up paddling, on a board, like a really big surfboard." I couldn't wait to try it!

From then on, we started paddling. We'd paddle in the early morning fog, under the midday sun, deep into fiery sunsets and beneath the rising moon. We'd paddle on bays, backwaters, harbors, the ocean, and even in the town pond! We paddled in bikinis and wetsuits, workout gear, and even dry suits in freezing weather. The sport was very male-oriented, and we became known as "The Paddle Divas."

Wherever we paddled, people who saw us wanted to join us and try this cool-looking sport. We spent most of our days loading up as many boards and paddles as could fit into Gina's truck and driving to a pristine bay. In no time, lessons became regularly scheduled and her clientele was built. Paddling was my escape from my chaotic and challenging (and often heartbreaking) life off the board. The lessons and

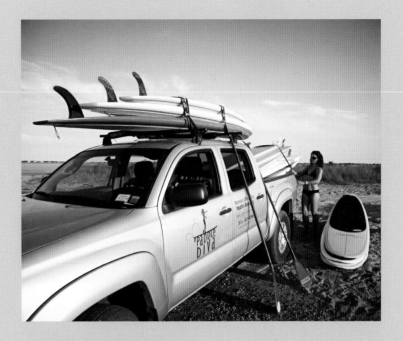

on-board fitness classes we created, the races we started competing in...for me, they were truly an extension of *freedom*. On my board, on the water, I felt transformed into a kind of superwoman—strong, in control, happy, fulfilled with my stressful life oceans away.

Something magical happens for me on a paddleboard. There is something about being on the water, about *floating*, that makes it so unlike anything else. I have to adapt to whatever Mother Nature presents me that day. Whether floating along in a glassy, protected bay or constantly falling off my board while paddling a downwinder on a choppy ocean, pushing myself to do sprints and work out on my board or challenging myself on a ten-mile distance paddle, it's always the same feeling at its core: I feel myself being fully present. Present with my surroundings, and mostly, present with myself. Paddling requires balance and steadfast attention, but once I settle into myself on the board, it feels more like meditation. When I paddle, I feel released. I feel free.

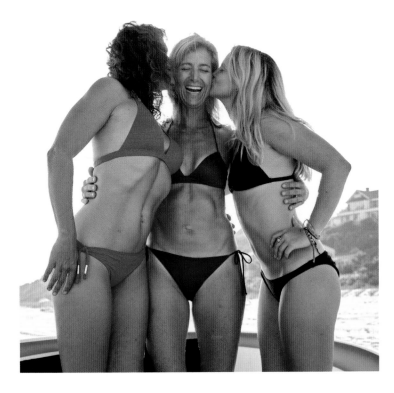

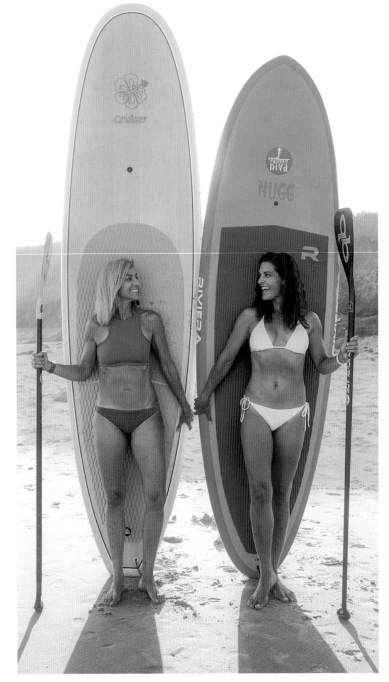

and so free as the two of us used to paddle and explore areas way beyond our skill set; we were driven by such determination and positivity. Whenever things got tough, we always made it back to shore. She learned then and applied to her journey with breast cancer the power of positivity to drive a positive end result!

So much of SUP is mental. I always say, if you have the willingness to try, you can SUP and succeed. You have to be positive and really want to try it and not worry about negative things you imagine could happen: that you'll fall in, that you'll hit your head, that you'll drown, or become so tired you won't make it back to shore. At the Paddle for Pink on that warm, windy day, my team of ten was filled with so many fears! We just had to all overcome these fears on land, get on our boards, paddle the course, cross the finish line and then *vavoom*: We will have proven to ourselves we could do it.

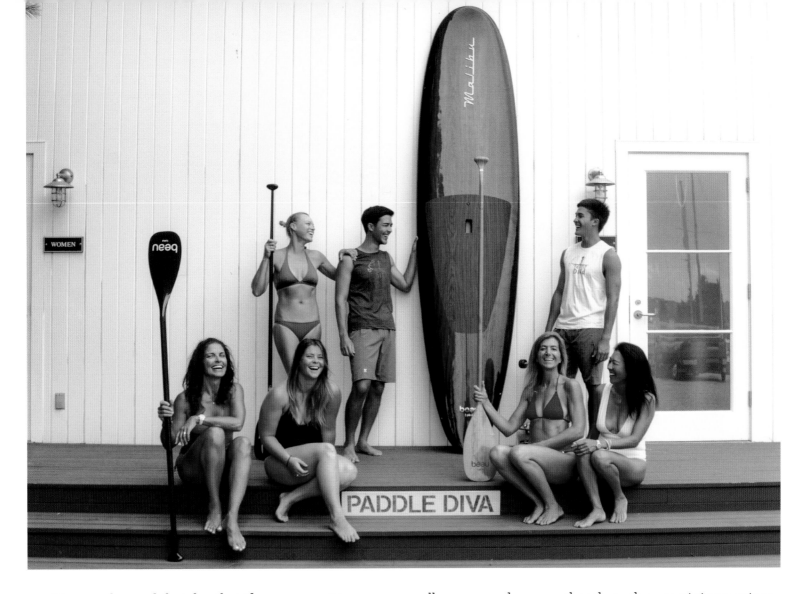

My team learned that day that if you are positive on the water during the race, you will be positive during the very next challenge you face. You will take this achievement of paddling in cloudy, rough conditions in the Paddle for Pink and apply it to the next challenge. It may be something that once felt so hard and now, because you have done something so remarkable on a board and achieved success, nothing will stop you if you keep yourself positive.

At the awards ceremony after the race, we all felt so energized and positive with a true sense of what it felt like to share this positivity with everyone. As a team, we all encouraged one another through our training sessions. We supported one another with cheers as we passed one another on the water. We hugged and supported other racers. We spent the day knowing that we as a group spread our positive energy from the pull of each stroke, building our cores from the inside out! We learned that the entire group of racers raised $1.4 million to help find a cure for breast cancer that day. It was one of the most powerful days for me as a Diva. I learned that positivity is contagious and just a little bit goes a long, long way. Much like the pull of a paddle as you glide through the water.

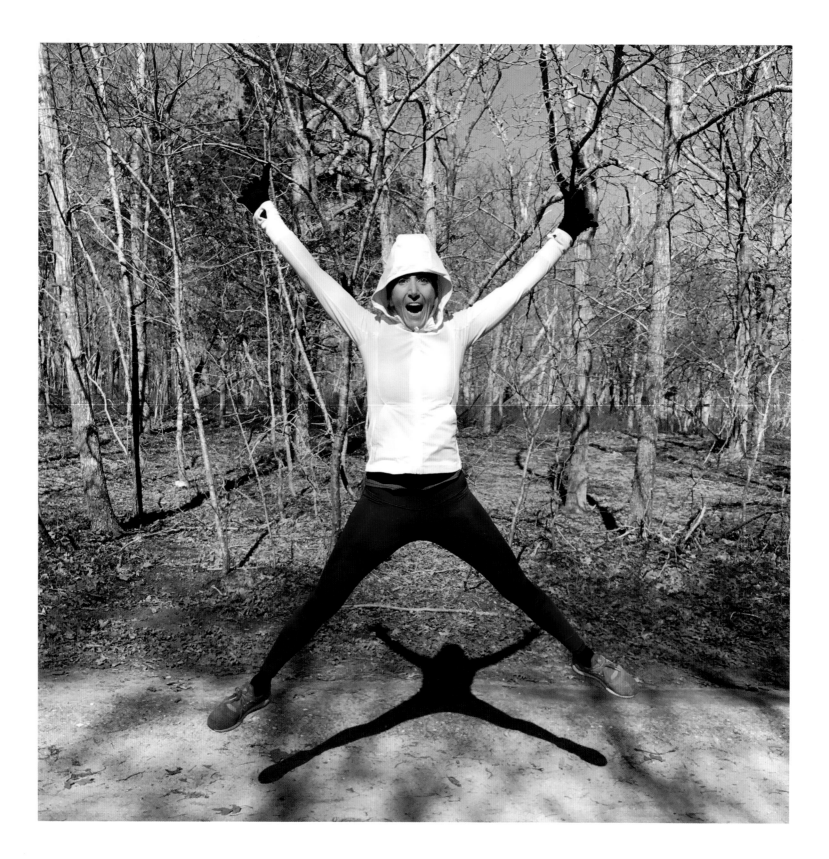

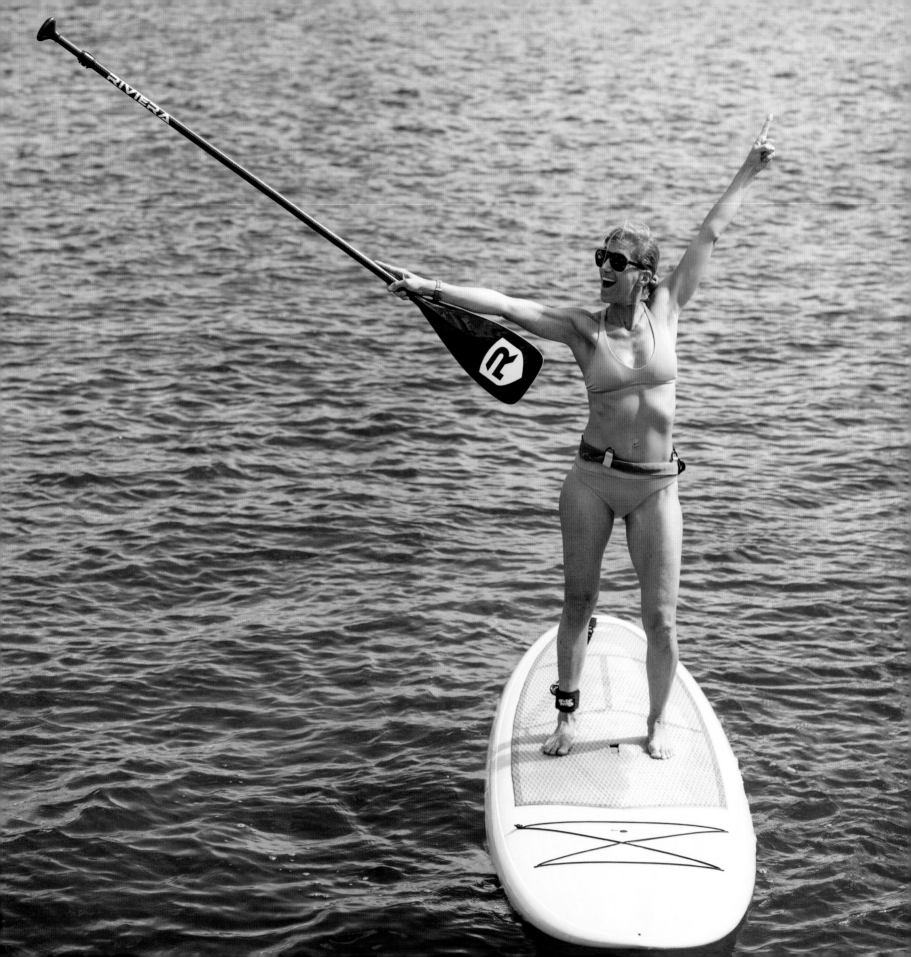

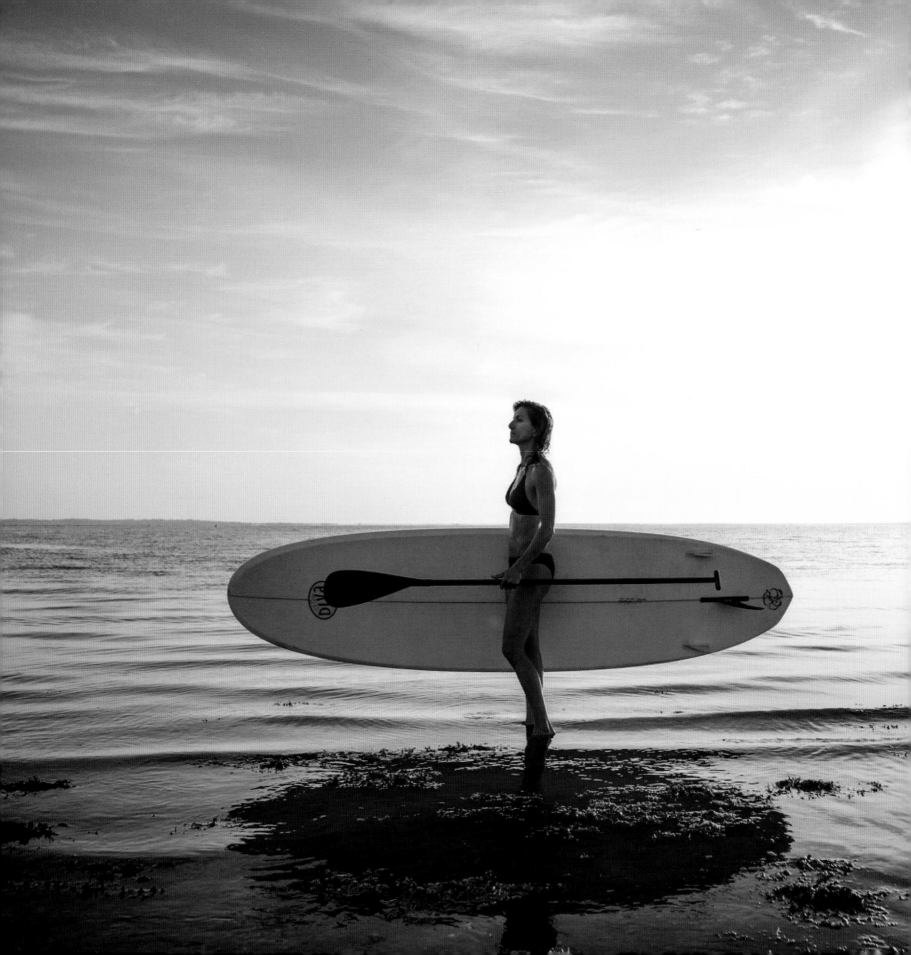

Be Open to the Outcome

The Hamptons are lined with hundreds of miles of calm, secluded bays, far away from the roar of the Atlantic Ocean. These little enclaves that dot the shores are so welcoming that they call to paddlers like the sirens of the sea. This paradise is my classroom. One warm and very windy day, I met my students at Haven's Beach. We were doing a paddle stroke clinic to help them go faster on the water.

"Today," I began the lesson, "we are going to practice stroke repetitions. Your top arm will come across your centerline, and you will twist your hip slightly to the opposite rail of the board. When you plant your paddle, you almost allow your body to fall on it but you don't fall in; the paddle braces you as catch the blade and pull it through the water." We all tried this movement on land and then I went on to teach, "If you fall, you're not failing. Falling will

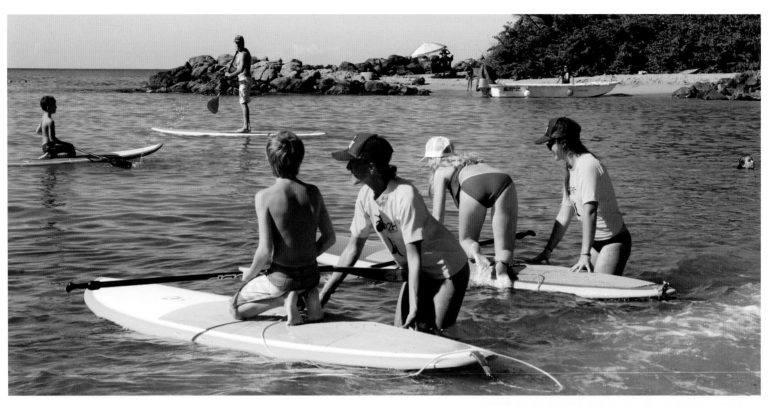

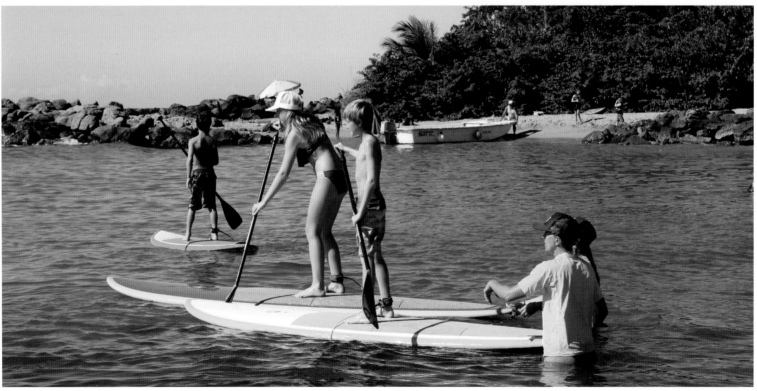

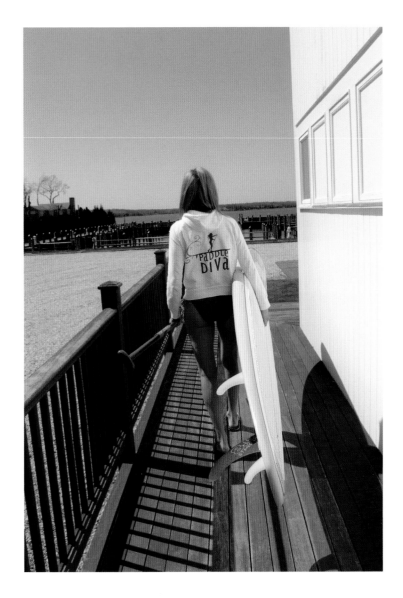

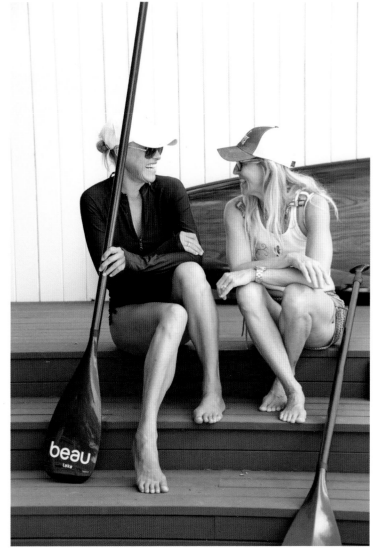

show me you are succeeding. You need to fall sometimes just to see how far you needed to lean out over the side or not; that's how you can gauge the motion and learn." This particular group was very focused on racing. "The same goes for racing. You have to completely distance yourself from any outcome you expect on the water and allow yourself to let go and let the water and the waves guide you in your success. Leave yourself open and available to an outcome that you can't see coming, often it is victory."

I teach beginners at this same beach in Sag Harbor due to its stillness. As you do when teaching a child to ride a bike, I will often hold the back of their boards steady until they are able to get their bearings. When I have these students standing on their boards and ready to launch, I consider that a great success. They are trying something new. My definition of success in SUP is often very different from my students'. For many, falling into the water is the worst thing that can happen to them on a

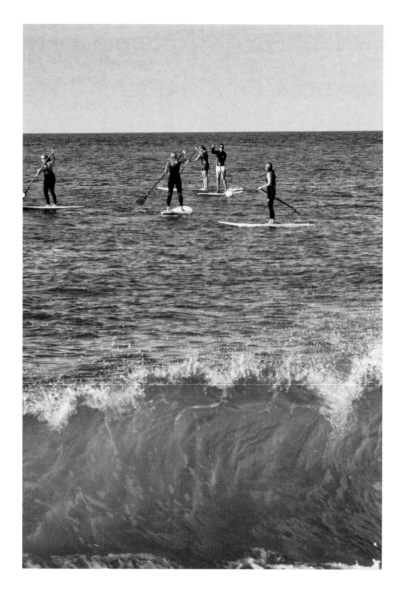

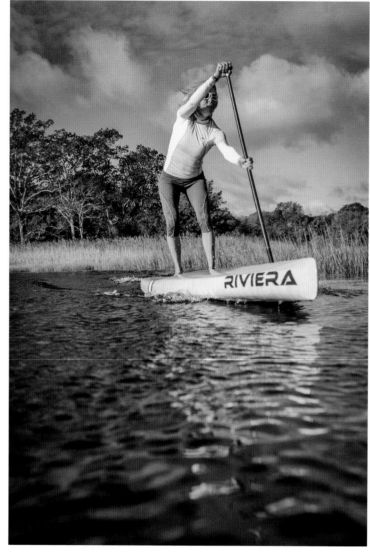

paddle excursion. They equate falling with failure. I like to remind them that success can take a multitude of shapes and forms on the water.

A lot of my students laugh when I say, "You have to be good at falling." Falling is actually a step in the learning process. When you fall in, you have to fall away from the board, in a starfish formation, body flat while still holding on to your paddle and keeping it away from you. We need everyone who learns how to paddle to do this at some

point, so when my beginners fall right away, we've gotten that over with and now we can move on to learning more moves. When someone who falls really feels downtrodden, I always stress that he or she actually has gone from a kneeling position to standing upright, which for many is an accomplishment in itself.

Stacey first came to me as a student, and over the past nine years has become a true Diva in her own right. She has taken the instructor certification course with me that

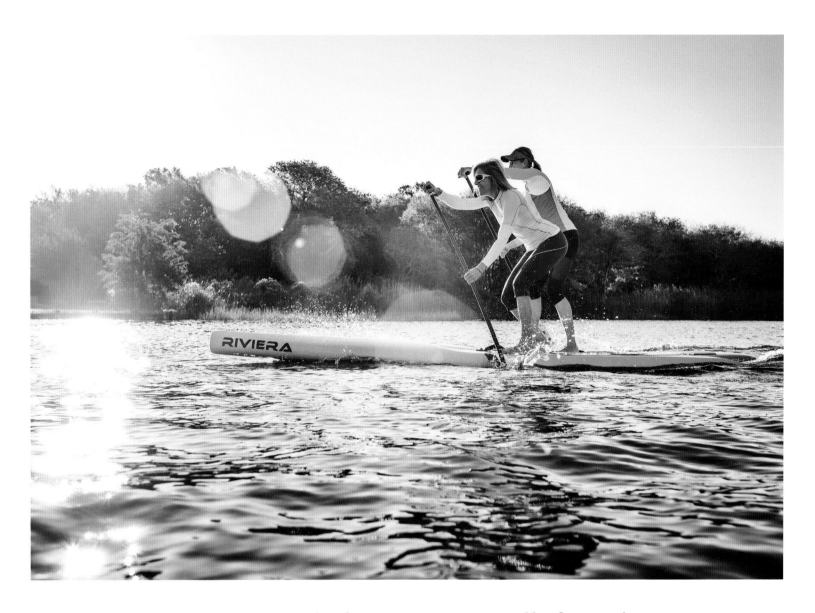

I am qualified to lead through the Academy of Surfing Instructors, a world-recognized leader in professional training and credentials for SUP. From the moment I met Stacey on this very same beach in Sag Harbor in 2010, I have always admired her ability to be in the moment. She has learned through her yoga practice and hours of training on the water to release all expectations before she sets out on the water.

Stacey joined her first race, the Great Peconic Race, in 2013; it raised money to help clean the bays of harmful algae. I was thrilled when she registered, but on the day of the race the winds where strong and none of us really knew what we were getting ourselves into. She was on her own SUP board, one that was stable, but on this day we all spent plenty of time in the water crawling back on the boards, popping up and continuing the race cadence.

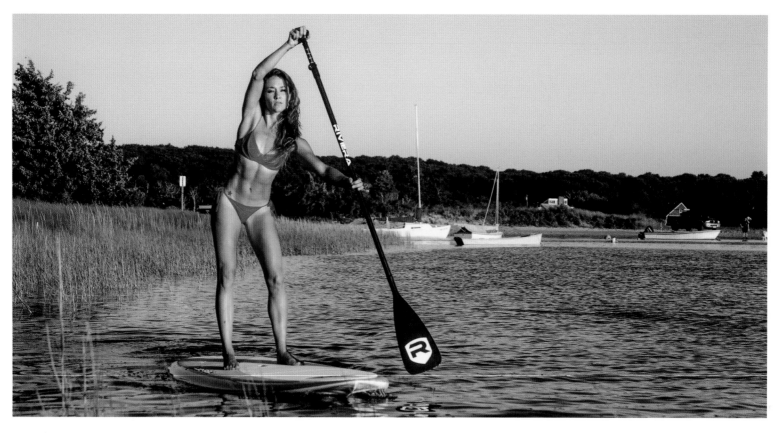

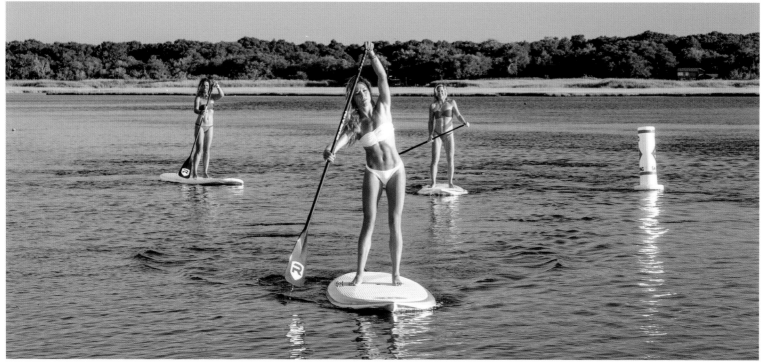

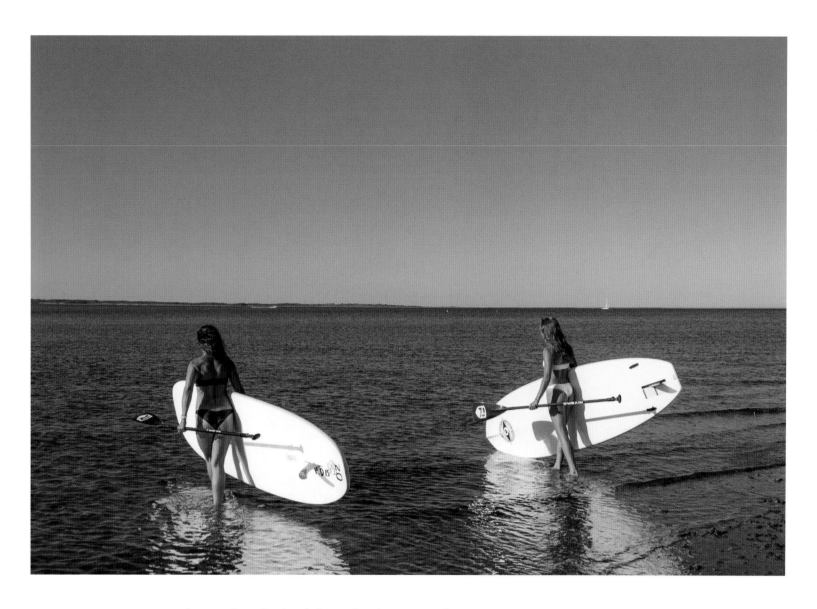

Stacey was a trooper, and even though she did not finish in the front of the pack and steadily held up the rear, she completed the race and felt so accomplished with just that—finishing the race, even though she almost came in last!

For many this experience would have been a bitter disappointment, but Stacey crossed that finish line beaming! Fundamentally, she was just proud of herself for even entering the race. Her success had less to do with winning, or even placing, than with her pure enjoyment of the experience. Stacey has since gone on to participate in many races because they are fun for her. She loves to race, and winning or losing makes no difference. She has released her ego from the outcome. Stacey has continued her journey in the SUP wellness world and has moved on to become one of Paddle Diva's lead SUP fitness instructors, getting as many credentials as she can acquire to hone her skills. She has become a barre

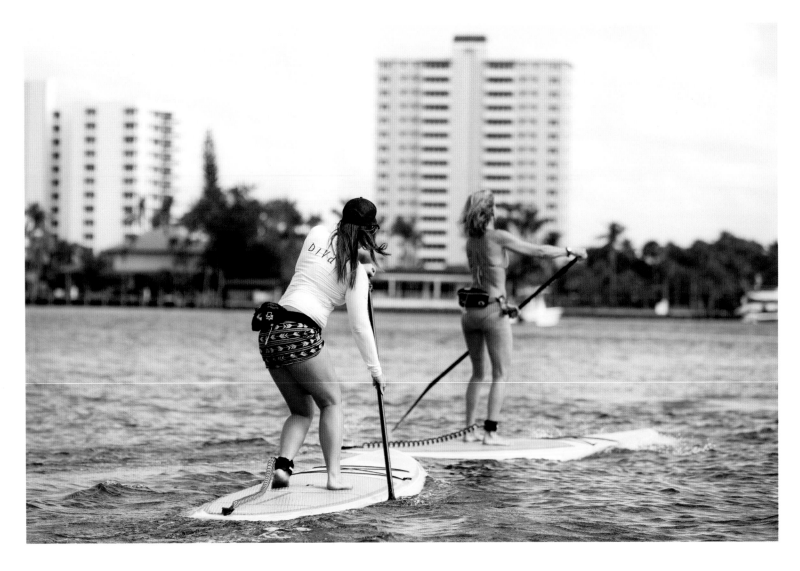

instructor through exhale spa's forty-hour teacher training. Stacey continues to take certification classes and teach fitness, completely unattached to the outcome but enjoying the path to get there!

In my everyday life, I see success and failure as nearly equal. Something good always comes out of a success, but something good *can* also come from failure—if you disconnect from your expectations and allow the positive to materialize. Most people, however, are so afraid to fail that they actually become an obstacle to their own success. I find the success within an experience, even if it didn't play out the way I expected.

In 2014, I had a situation in which my presence in what was a sleepy, underutilized private marina suddenly became a problem for two of my neighbors. They felt that the zoning for a marina did not apply to a paddleboard business. I was operating out of the little office inside the main building and on the beach that flanked either side of the marina enclosure. I had to endure a two-year process of hearings and public meetings to end up with

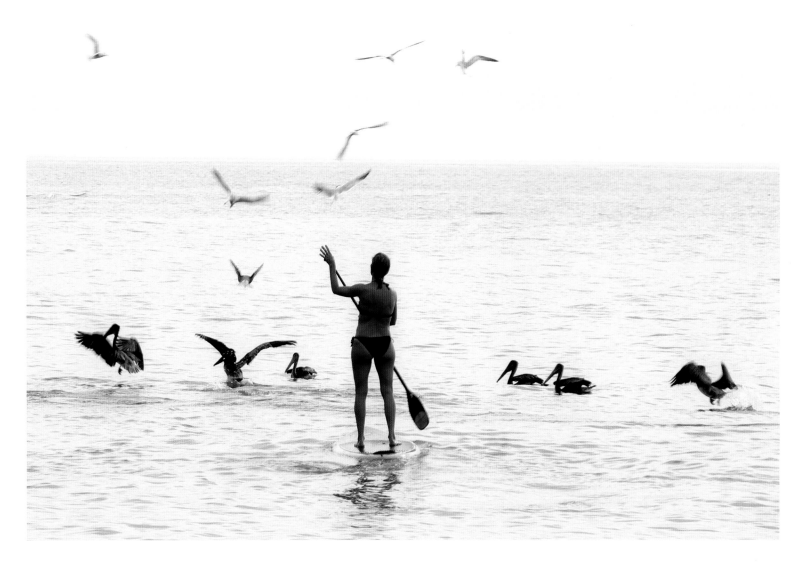

an ambiguous decision from the zoning board that led to the probability that my non-motorized, environmentally friendly, family-oriented business might have to close! I embarked on a long legal process of suing the town's ruling in what is called an Article 78. I did this knowing that the outcome might not be in my favor. But I pursued this course because I believed that what I was doing was for the good of the residents of Long Island's East End and was good for the environment, as my business opens up students' minds to pay attention to the environment

that so needs our attention. I did not care about the potential outcome of the judge's ruling; I cared about the journey and knew that no matter what, Divas would always have a place to paddle. Paddle Diva would never go away.

On a hot summer morning in 2016, the judge ruled from the bench in oral arguments, in Paddle Diva's favor—a rare occurrence. With the slam of his gavel, the stroke of his pen, and the intelligence and fairness of his ruling, I remained in my precious headquarters.

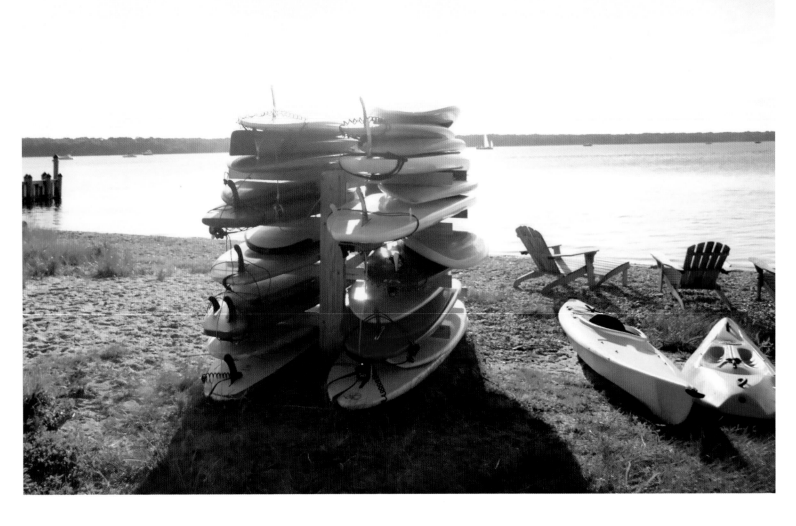

The outcome was what I could have only dreamed of, and the journey has made me a better businesswoman, more assured of myself and my beliefs.

Following this historic win in the state supreme court, I began to reflect on when I started the business. I had not really been thinking back then if it would fail or succeed. I knew I wanted to do something that would allow people into my world, to experience a sport that felt difficult to learn, and to make it truly accessible to all. I had the journey picked out, and the outcome, whether the business was going to boom or go bust, never crossed my mind. I was open to the outcome. Just weeks after the judge overturned the town's zoning decision to not allow me to operate at my marina location, as I took my team through the lesson, they shed their fear of falling. We all pushed hard and one by one fell into the cooling waters off Sag Harbor bay. We all knew that falling was only one part of this amazing journey we were taking on that day.

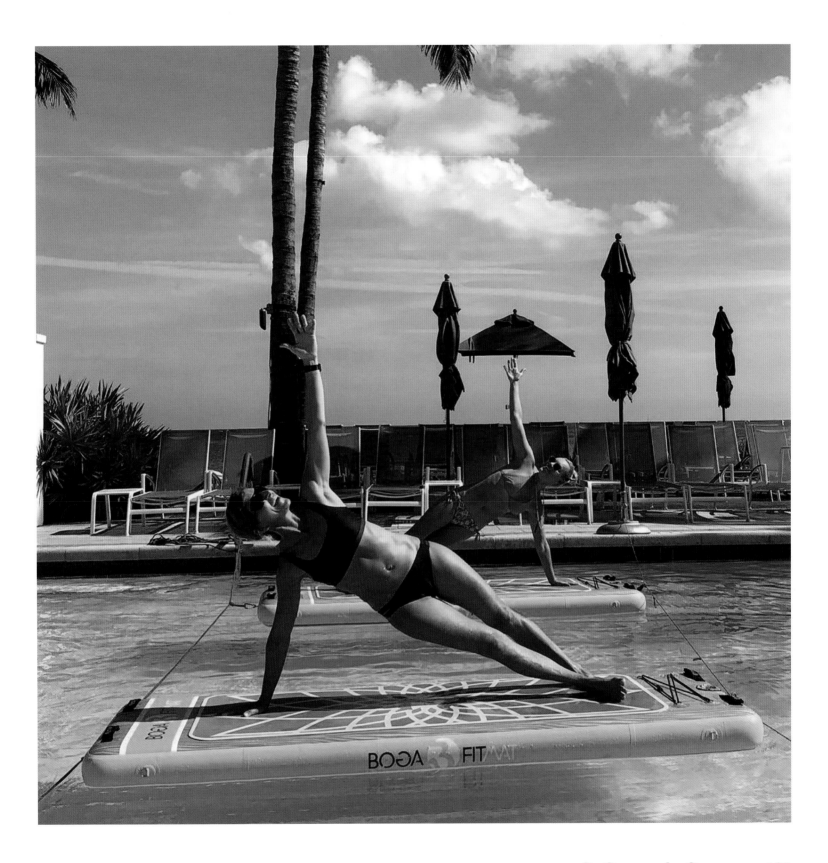

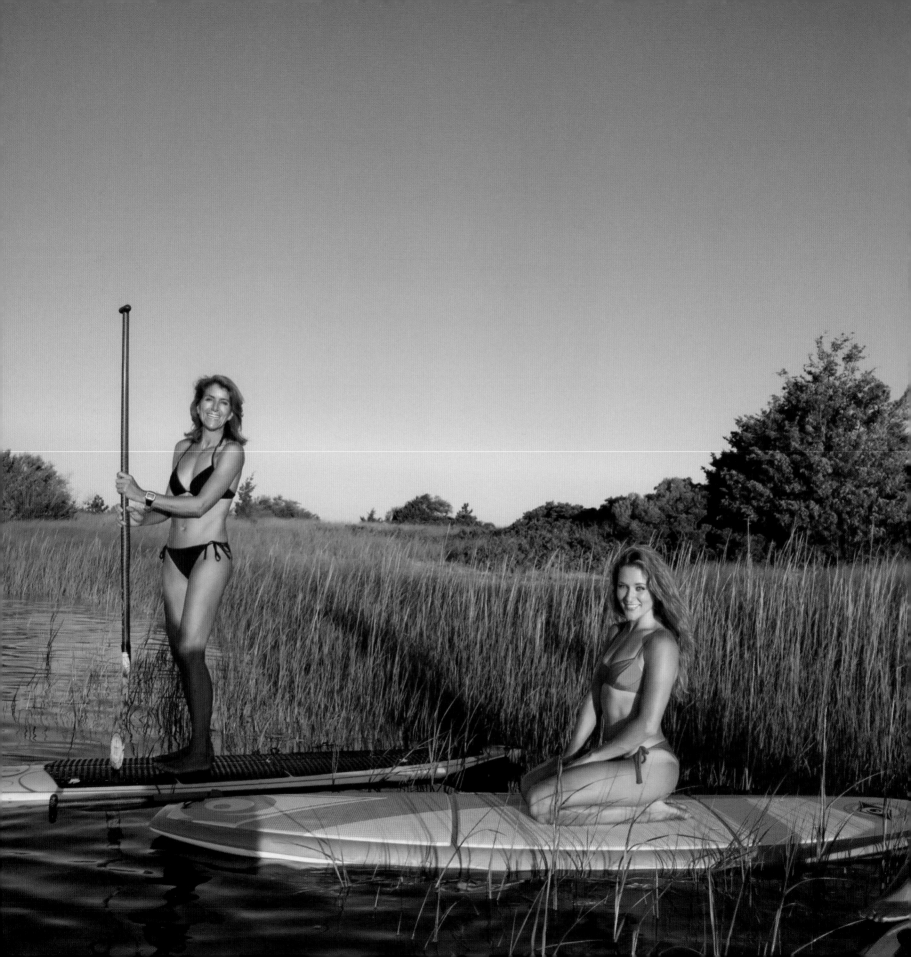

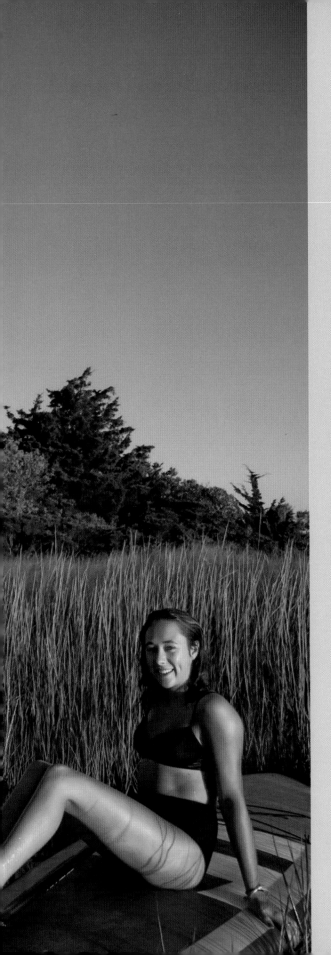

Laugh Every Day, Smile Every Hour

"Today we are getting out of the gym and into nature," I tell my students at the beginning of the combination paddle + barre event we offer throughout the summer in partnership with Elisabeth Halfpap from exhale spa. Elisabeth exudes positive energy with her smiling blue eyes that invite you into whatever she's doing. She's one of those unique people you meet who are always beaming with happiness. She loves this class, paddling, and being outdoors as much as I do. For over five years, Paddle Diva and exhale spa have been teaming up to offer our students a SUP barre experience. This is a paddle class that combines the core work required to paddle effectively with an intense workout on the paddleboard that uses an adapted series of barre moves to give our students the most complete workout.

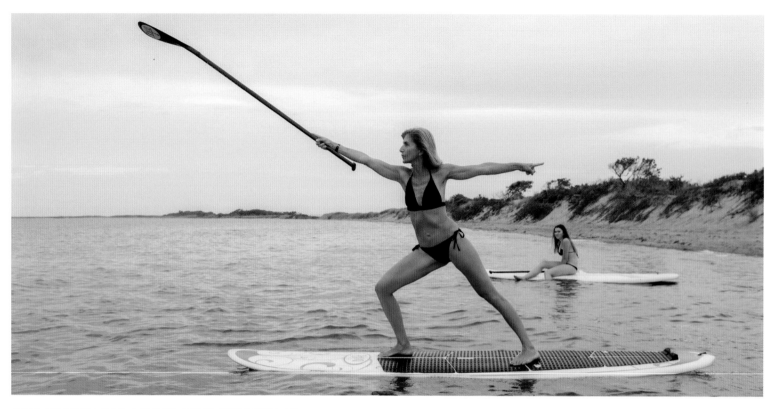

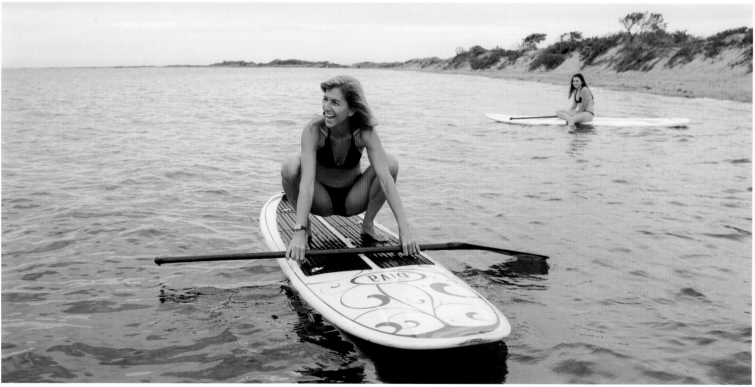

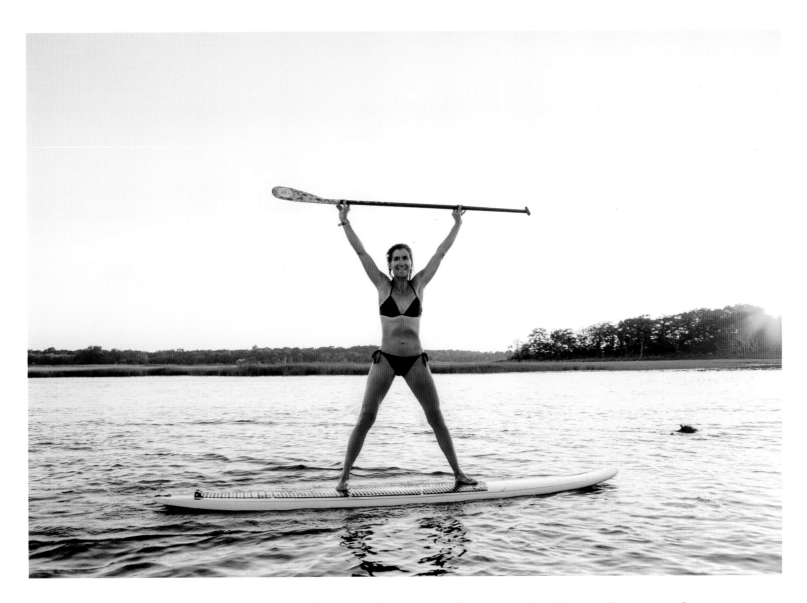

In the first twenty minutes, students do a fast-paced paddle, then we anchor our boards and do a modified barre sequence on the board. We do planks, push-ups, and curls—we even use our paddles as our barres. It may sound daunting, but it is really fun. It's a class filled with lightness and laughter because working out outside is so freeing. It's also a great opportunity to introduce more people to the wonders of our pristine environment and what we can all do to protect it!

After a quick land lesson, this group of twenty men and woman were ready to set off. Elisabeth's energy and excitement are infectious as she got the class launched alongside me. In ankle-deep water, we all kneeled on the soft deck pads of our boards. David, who was over six feet tall and part of a group of friends who all joined this class together, was eager to get going to sweat out his hangover. As he rose quickly to his feet, he locked his knees and the board started to wobble. He quickly looked down and at

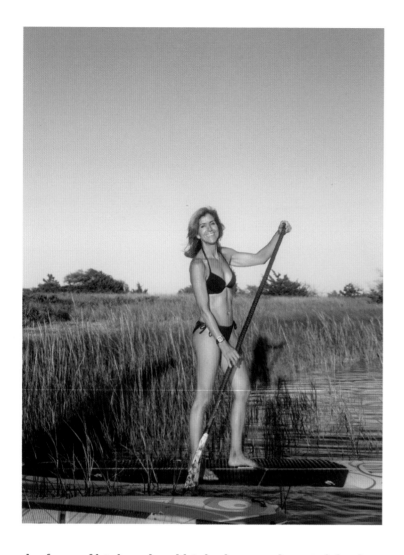

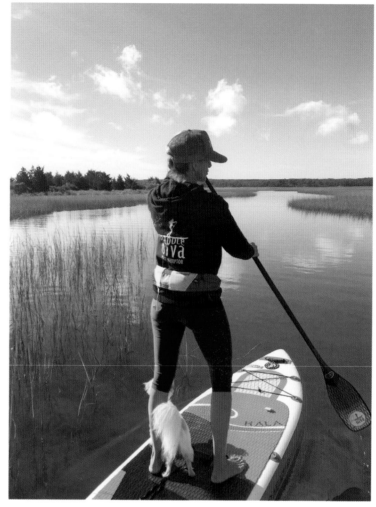

the front of his board and his body started to pitch back and forth like a dinghy caught in a typhoon. It was almost too comical for even me to keep a straight face. While his friends tried unsuccessfully to hold back giggles and laughter, I regained my composure and paddled over to him quickly. "Look up at the horizon," I told him as we made eye contact. "Breathe out and put your paddle in the water. Stand tall and *smile*!" He picked up these cues quickly. His brow furrowed and his eyes brightened. He smiled and looked out at the horizon. He started laughing in relief, and then just like that he was back in control.

He plunged his paddle deep in the water, till the blade was submerged and pulled it back to his body, which propelled him and his board through the water. Like a rocket he was off and leading the group. Feeling the pressure to succeed now, the group regained composure and they all started the paddle sprints. Elisabeth, who was enjoying her moments on the water, gleefully called out to David, "Abs in. Hold your core and breathe." As we all paddled I pointed out the phragmites and the eel grass and spotted oysters resting gently on the seabed below. Oysters help to flush out impurities in the waters and

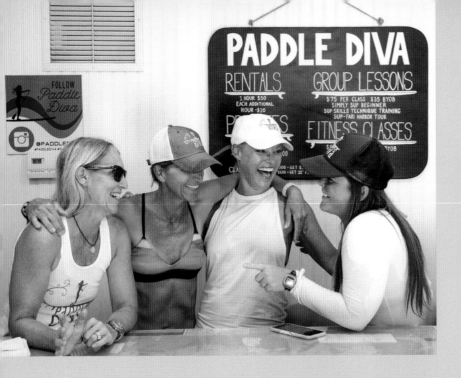

Paddle Diva Frequently Asked Questions

By Amy Worthington, Paddle Diva instructor

In the heat of the summer months, if you dial (631) 329-2999, you will be greeted with a joyful and enthusiastic, "Paddle Diva; this is Amy!" It's like the song of a bird, reaching through the phone and beckoning you to smile before you continue. The age-old adage "There's no such thing as a silly question" definitely applies here, but there are some common questions that put a smile on all of our faces.

"I know you're called Paddle Diva, but do you also teach guys?"

With a hint of a giggle, we always respond, "Of course, we teach guys! Paddle Diva is for everyone." We understand where the confusion comes from. The name was inspired by a conversation Gina had with her husband, an avid waterman. When talking about Gina's vision to bring paddleboarding from the ocean to the bay and make her lifestyle of balance and wellness more accessible to the masses, he jokingly commented, "Well, you should just call it Paddle Diva." The name, and the intention, stuck. We're not all divas in the conventional sense, but everyone has at least a little Paddle Diva in them.

"What is the age restriction for SUP? Can I sign my child up for a lesson?"

We get this question all the time. The truest answer is that every child is different. Each has different strengths and fears, and a different attention span and learning style. At Paddle Diva, the most important aspects of a successful kid lesson are keeping them in their comfort zone, having fun, and never allowing them to have a bad or unsafe experience on the water, all while empowering them to paddle their boards with strength and independence.

"What should I wear? Do I need a wetsuit or water shoes?"

Wear whatever makes you comfortable! On hot days, when the sun is out, if you're comfortable with your bathing suit, wear just that, but any quick-drying, non-cotton athletic wear will do. The most important thing is that you feel comfortable and confident. You will see Gina from sunup to sundown in her bikini, while others are out on the water in workout pants and a tank top. We do encourage rash guards or some kind of sun protection if you have fair skin, and a hat you don't mind getting wet. And, if you're bringing your favorite sunglasses, make sure you have a Croakie—a strap that attaches your sunglasses to your head so you don't lose them to the ocean!

We have a fantastic website, with all the information you might need about Paddle Diva, our lifestyle, and the types of lessons we provide, but we do answer the phone night and day to answer any and all questions you may have. People know they can get ahold of us to ask about paddling conditions for the day anywhere in the Hamptons. They call to ask what new board or paddle they should order, or to let us know they will be stopping by for a paddle. We always answer with a smile.

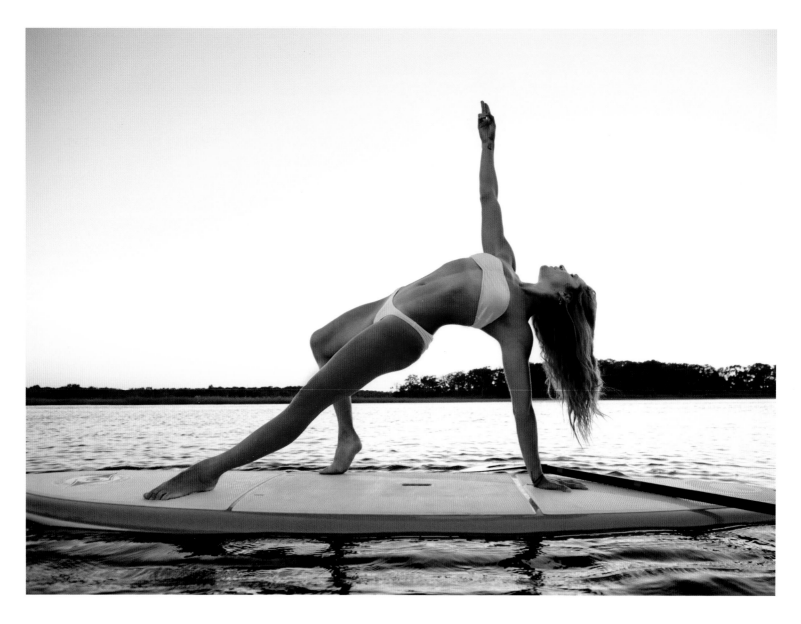

keep the bay clean and healthy. I pointed out the incoming tide, bringing us fresh seawater from the ocean just outside the harbor.

Smiles and laughter make such a difference on the water and even in a barre studio. If there are two people on the planet that exemplify this, they are Elisabeth and Fred, business partners and spouses for over thirty-five years. They know how to create a nurturing, joyful environment with students. They both beam with positive energy. Whenever I teach with Elisabeth and the wind, weather, or tides have an impact on our class (making it difficult but never impossible), we always have the same exact mantra: "We'll make this work." And we always do. Studies have shown that smiling makes the brain emit feel-good neurotransmitters, such as dopamine, endorphins, and serotonin. This not only relaxes your body and

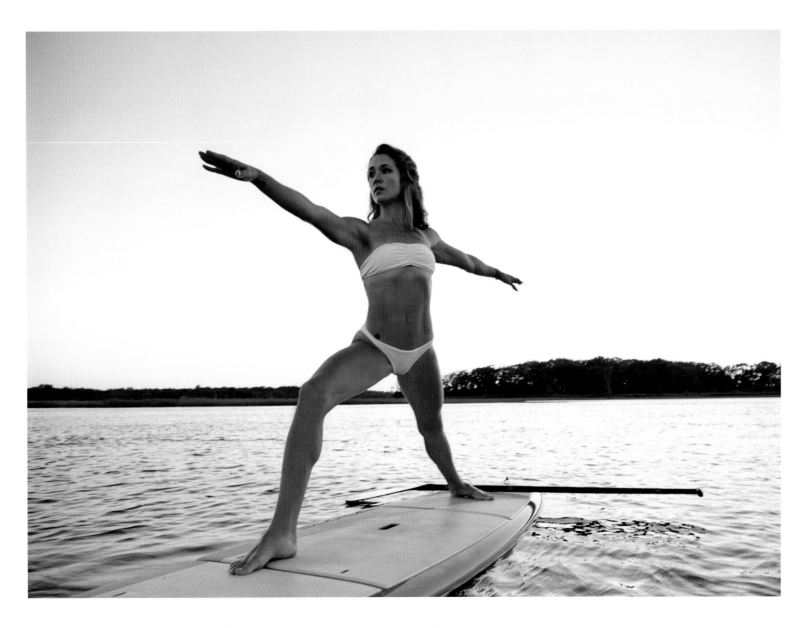

gives you a sense of general well-being, but it can also lower your heart rate and blood pressure. So, it can be a big help to people who are dealing with a seemingly tippy board, nervousness about trying something new, their perceived "bad balance," or even terror of the water. A smile gives me a true sense of amusement.

I watch beginners get from a kneeling to a standing position. As they stand up on their boards, their shoulders will slowly inch up towards their ears and their mouths will settle into tight, straight line. I quickly tell them to smile and to breathe. Then as the water gently washes up on the top of the board and cools their feet and they find their balance by looking at the horizon, they start to feel the rush of excitement as their boards move forward with each stroke. The smiles that appear on their faces last the entire paddle and take them through the entire day!

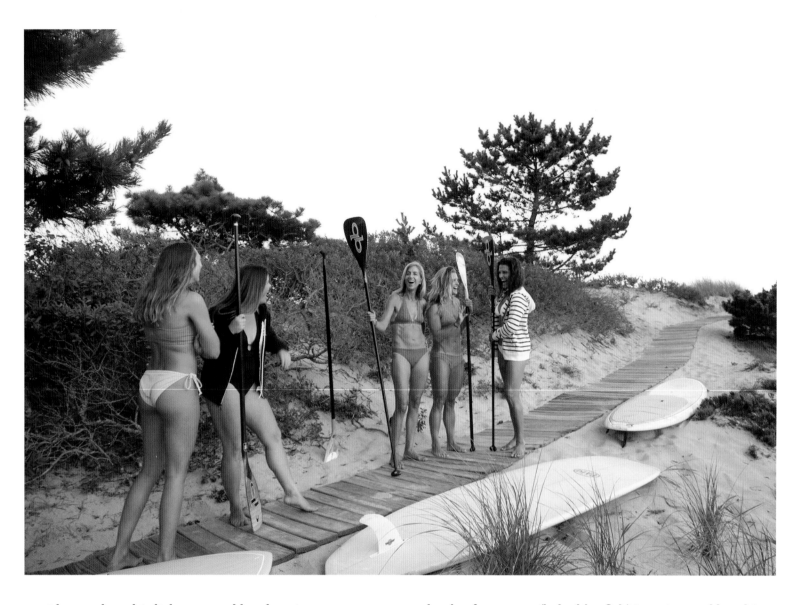

I have taken this lightness and laughter into my own world starting very recently, when I became involved with many groups to raise awareness of the need to restore our waters: fresh water and sea water. My smile and joyous laughter come naturally when I see a pod of dolphins off in the distance, or if a sea turtle peeks its head out to say hello before darting back down to the deep, or if a curious manatee follows me, enjoying the shade my board makes in the clear waters, or when I see

schools of snappers (baby bluefish) jumping and breaking the surface so it almost looks like it's raining fish for a moment, or times like this past summer when I was honored to have a mother and father swan raise their cygnet on my beach. I have fallen in love with the environment, and this drives me to have my students deepen their understanding of why it is so important to take small steps to start preserving and protecting our precious and delicate world.

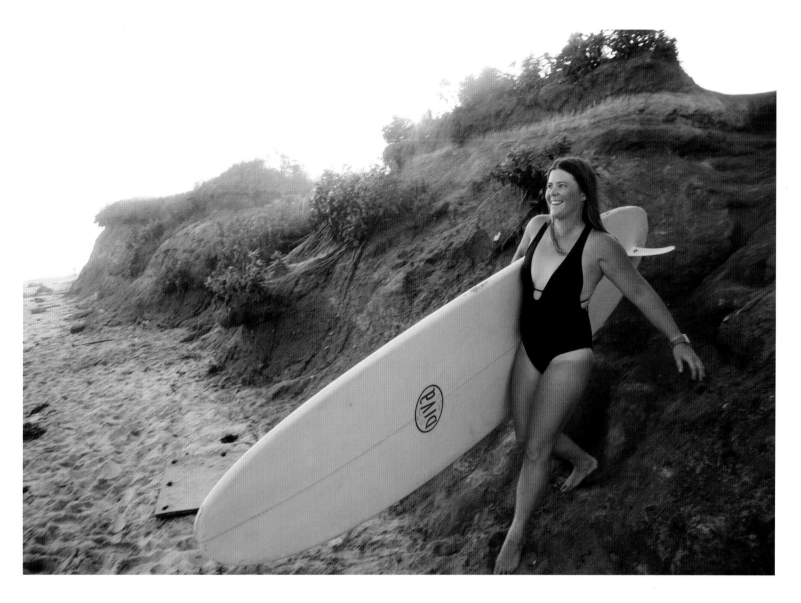

Like our own bodies, the oceans need rest and plenty of attention. They need to smile. I sometimes use my time on the board to share this with my students and help them make the mind-body-earth connection, as I call it. If we can all come together to keep the abundance the earth has provided for millennia and we do things to help take care of our precious planet, it will bring a smile to our faces and joy to our lives, just knowing we are contributing. As a friend once said to me, "If Mother Earth smiles, we smile along with her." The power of this lies in the proof. The next time you are standing near a waterway, look out as far as your eyes can see. Let your face relax. Feel the earth smiling down on you as your eyes follow the smile shape of the circumference of the earth. You will smile right back at her. And you will carry this smile along with you for the rest of your day.

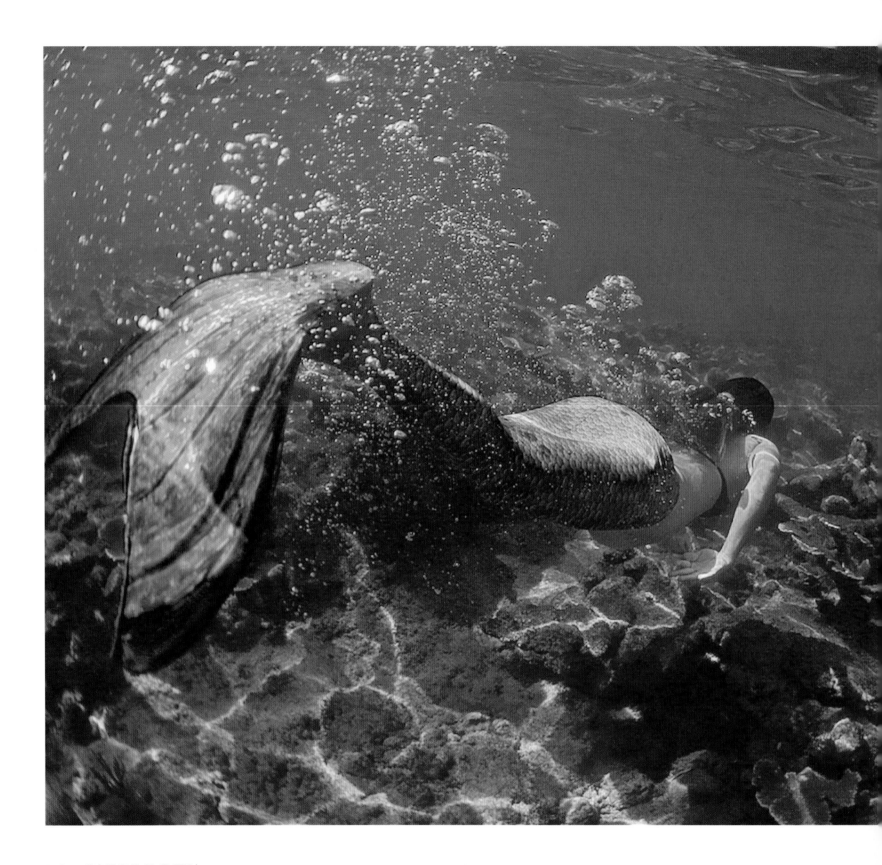

Afterword

During the summer of 2010, I was in search of a teacher who could get me out on the water on the East End of Long Island. I'd tried surfing but wanted something more meditative. I also wanted a family-friendly sport that would allow us to observe the beauty of the area's bays and waterways, the architecture of the great homes along the coast of Long Island, as well as the brackish ponds along the ocean where bird life was abundant. Luckily, I found Gina Bradley and her business Paddle Diva.

She turned up at my home with her big silver truck stacked high with paddles boards. I immediately fell in love with Gina's spirit: her entrepreneurial energy and genuine excitement to get people out on the water. "It's the best form of exercise," she told me, as we paddled out together the first time. "Plus, I love the sounds of water moving, the smell of salt water and the negative ions that are produced by the sea will elevate your mood. Sounds contrary but it's not, I promise!"

We spent ten years paddling together. Being on the water nourished a lot of conversions about ocean concerns and the need to wake people up to the beauty and fragility of our natural ecosystems. As a board member of Oceana, I not only wanted to protect our oceans but also take time to deepen my connection to them. I was so inspired by my time with Gina that I brought paddleboards to Maine where I continue to paddle with my children and husband around Seal Harbor. We all get a topnotch core workout as well as a unique perspective of the various sailboats, lobster, and picnic boats on moorings in the harbor. I wear my Paddle Diva sweatshirt or rash guard and am reminded of Gina and the joy she's brought to my family.

Not only is Gina a wonderful teacher, she's also a dedicated ocean advocate and conservation leader, or what I like to call a Mermaid Ambassador of the Hamptons. In 2012, we collaborated on a film I produced and directed linking the myth of the mermaid to ocean health (http://www.missionofmermaids.com). In it, Gina explains how each person can play a part in reducing negative impacts to our oceans by altering their daily actions.

Mother, activist, conservationist, entrepreneur, Gina Bradley knows a lot. And the lessons embodied in her book can be applied to anybody looking for exercise, a spiritual connection to the sea, heightened awareness, a slower pace and deeper breathing, magical moments in the here and now as well as getting to know ourselves better. All of which help us handle the changing currents and winds that are intrinsic to this journey of life.

—*Susan Rockefeller*

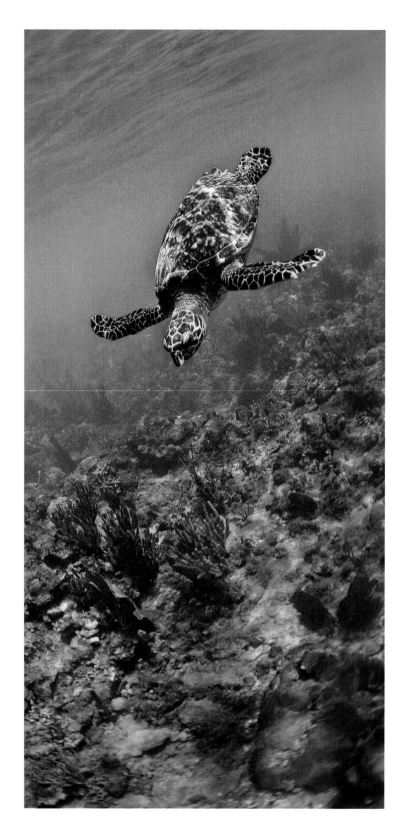

Causes and Businesses

4 OCEAN

This global movement focuses on actively removing trash from the ocean and coastlines while inspiring individuals to work together for cleaner oceans, one pound at a time.

www.4ocean.com

ACADEMY OF SURFING INSTRUCTORS (ASI)

ASI is the world's leading stand-up paddle accreditation and training organization. It provides services to SUP schools, instructors, and the general public.

www.academyofsurfing.com/stand-up-paddle

CORNELL COOPERATIVE EXTENSION

Cornell Cooperative Extension puts knowledge to work in pursuit of economic vitality, ecological sustainability, and social well-being.

www.ccesuffolk.org/marine

EXHALE

Exhale spa is one part fitness, one part spa, and all parts total well-being experience.

www.exhalespa.com

GROUP FOR THE EAST END

Group for the East End protects and restores the environment of eastern Long Island through professional advocacy and education. It inspires people to embrace a conservation ethic and to take action in their local communities.

www.groupfortheeastend.org

THE GREAT PECONIC RACE

The GPR was created to let paddlers experience the beauty of the Peconic Bay and to challenge their will to withstand whatever Mother Nature throws at them, and to raise money for the Cornell Cooperative Extension Marine Program, which helps to save our waters.

www.greatpeconicrace.com

HAMPTONS PARTY AND PADDLE FOR PINK

The Hamptons Party and Paddle for Pink together form an annual event benefiting the Breast Cancer Research Foundation (BCRF).

www.hamptonspaddleforpink.org

MUSINGS

Founded by Susan Rockefeller, Musings is a bi-monthly newsletter and digital magazine that curates ideas and innovations that pave the way for a more sustainable future.

www.musingsmag.com

MISSION OF MERMAIDS

Mission of Mermaids (MOM) is a short film celebrating director Susan Rockefeller's relationship with the ocean. It's both a poetic ode to the seas and a plea for their protection.

www.missionofmermaids.com

OCEANA

Oceana is dedicated to protecting and restoring the world's oceans on a global scale.

www.oceana.org

PECONIC BAYKEEPER

Peconic Baykeeper is an organization dedicated to protecting and restoring Long Island's swimmable, drinkable, and fishable waters.

www.peconicbaykeeper.org

SURFRIDER FOUNDATION

The Surfrider Foundation is a grassroots non-profit environmental organization that works to protect and preserve the world's oceans, waves, and beaches.

www.surfrider.org

TOWN OF EAST HAMPTON SHELLFISH HATCHERY

The Aquaculture Department exists for the purpose of enhancing commercially valuable molluscan shellfish stocks in local waters.

www.ehamptonny.gov/149/aquaculture

XPT

XPT is an experience and a fitness vacation. Breathe, move, and recover with the XPT founders themselves, surf legend and innovator Laird Hamilton and former professional athlete Gabrielle Reece for an exclusive hands-on, three-day fitness vacation at an exclusive partnered resort.

www.xptlife.com

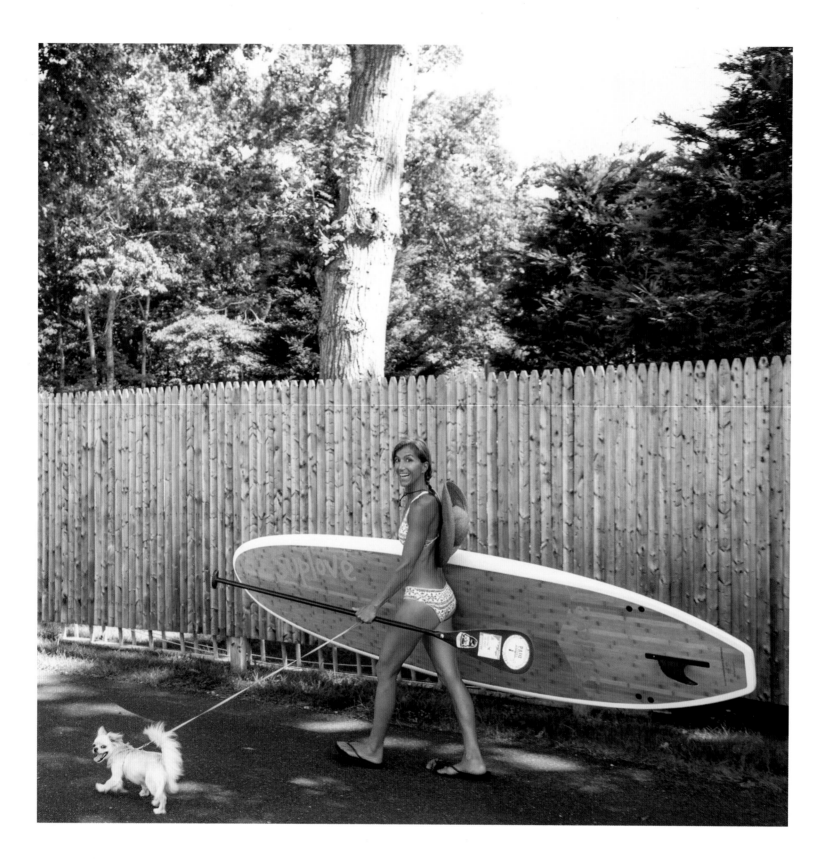

Contributing Photographers

I will forever be grateful to the women and men behind the lens. When I started Paddle Diva ten years ago, I built my website using the snapshots I had in my digital camera. It was a time that preceded the smart phone, Instagram, photo-driven websites, and social media. I quickly learned that the emotional and visual aspects of my stand-up paddling lifestyle had to be shot with a discerning and experienced eye. Over the past ten years, I have been accumulating shots, working with professionals who have done for Paddle Diva what I can now do for the world: make the stand-up paddling experience accessible to all!

Here is thanks to the amazing photographers whose breathtaking images have brought this book to life:

MICHAEL WILLIAMS

themichaelwilliams.com

BRIAN BLOOM

brianbloomphotographs.com

RACHEL TANNER

racheltannerphotography.com

ANGELO CORDERO

angelocordero.com/portfolio

ERIC STRIFFLER

ericstriffler.com

DURRELL GODFREY

East Hampton Star

JEAN HODGENS

jeanhodgens.com

EVENLY O'DOHERTY

evelynodoherty.com

NATE BEST

natebest.com

TONY ZACHAREK

instagram.com/tonyzphotos

Acknowledgments

I am grateful to so many people who have taken this ride with me. This book is more than what it seems. Paddle Diva is a ten-year living and breathing business that has touched so many lives, enriched my own, and become a movement. My gratitude will never stop. To anyone I may have forgotten to mention here, just know that if we have ever shared a smile or engaged in a conversation, I am thankful to you, and when we meet again, I will acknowledge you personally.

I am eternally thankful to my family. My mom, Lex Lalli, who always encouraged me to write and has never stopped believing in what I can do and pushing me to always do more. My father, Lou Lalli, who taught me to love the ocean at an early age when we started SCUBA diving together. My sister, Nica Lalli, and her husband, Greg Littleton, who were enormous sources of support and guidance when I needed it throughout the drafting of this book. My husband, Scott, who still has a file on my computer called "my hot husband" filled with shots of him riding giant waves I can only dream of charging. He was responsible for coming up with the name Paddle Diva and has been my utmost support while the business expanded. There are also, of course, Emma and James, who are my main motivating force in life and have truly tested the Guiding Principles and push me to live by what I have written!

I must thank all my Divas. Yes, my inner circle. The friends you'd want in your life raft should the ship ever go down. You know who you are, and I will always rely on you all. From photo shoots to paddle races, you have all been there for me and I for you when in need. Friendships forged with the commonality of a love for the ocean will last forever.

I want to recognize Ben Krupinski, posthumously. Ben helped me get on the map in the Hamptons by providing me a legitimate home base and paddle center in the Shagwong Marina. I still miss our morning coffee and walks down to Shagwong Beach. I must thank Susan and David Rockefeller, some of my very first clients in the summer of 2010, who so gently planted the seed of conservationism in my life and my business that has now grown into a lifelong mission.

To get this book done, it took so many people who believed in me. For this I thank Jasmyn Pizzimbono. You've been my advisor, business seer, and friend. Thank you for pushing me to do this. I am grateful to Emily Klein, who, with her talents of listening and penning, was able to craft a proposal that gave me the power to write in my own voice. I have to thank Amy Worthington for poring over thousands of photos while helping me put this book together and for tirelessly managing Paddle Diva.

This book would have never happened were it not for one of my student, Katherine Malloy, who so innocently mentioned that her husband was in publishing and maybe he and I should meet. Anthony Ziccardi and Post Hill Press are where my thankfulness pours out. Anthony, in less than one hour of talking, took me on and brought me into his world of publishing. I love my editor, Wenonah Hoye, who became an invaluable resource as I sent her pages and pages of my writing, for her sheer faith in my ability to get this done and done on time! Thank you to the entire Post Hill team—you are truly masters at merging the words and photography to bring my vision for this book to life.

I close with a final thank you to *you*, the reader of this book. We are now connected. You understand what it means to be a Diva living a balanced life. So, now that we know each other, come on down to one of our Paddle Diva centers and let's SUP. Let me show you the way!